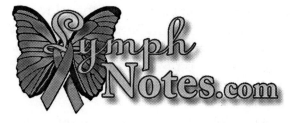

Reviewer comments:

A very encouraging book—like having your own therapist and a close friend along as you try new behaviors.
Claudia Kelsey

Empowering and practical, with exercises the reader can jump right into and know they are taking steps to help themselves. I love the emphasis throughout the book that the patient is in control.
Christine P. Thomas, MSPT, CLT-LANA

I learned from each part. I'm going to copy a few pages for my employer; I've asked my husband to read the section for him; my therapist wants a copy.
Pat Speckman

I found this book immediately comforting. Lymphedema can be isolating but this book helped me feel less alone. … I believe anyone with lymphedema or their loved ones will benefit from this book
Adrienne, recently diagnosed with lymphedema

A refreshing and inspiring journey through understanding and coping with lymphedema. … Readers will consult it frequently like a reference tool. Recommended for public libraries, consumer health libraries, and mental health professionals working in oncology.
Beth Hill, University of Idaho in Library Journal, October 2005

I think this book is very valuable and a great tool for healthcare professionals and patients alike. I hope it will help strengthen my relationship with my patients and the effectiveness of our work.
Doris Laing, LMBT, CLT-LANA

Helping us know how to provide for our own needs and to overcome the emotionally crippling results of lymphedema.
Karen Kohr-Blinn

This book is full of basic psychological truths which are insightful, constructive, and very helpful.
Judith Janaro Fabian, PhD, ABPP

Overcoming
the Emotional Challenges of
Lymphedema

Elizabeth McMahon, PhD

Lymph Notes
San Francisco

Overcoming the Emotional Challenges of Lymphedema
© 2005 by Lymph Notes

Lymph Notes
2929 Webster Street
San Francisco, CA 94123 USA
www.LymphNotes.com   sales@lymphnotes.com

ISBN 0-9764806-3-8
Library of Congress Control Number: 2005931782
Publishing history—first edition, printing 1.00

Cover pastel by Patty Rice, www.pattyrice.com

Foreword

When we were planning **Living Well With Lymphedema,** we knew that the emotional aspects of lymphedema were a major issue. After we asked Elizabeth McMahon to write a chapter on emotions we quickly learned that the topic was more complex than we had realized and that we had clearly found the right expert for this job. It also was painfully obvious that this important topic had never been fully explored in terms of understanding the issues and providing practical solutions.

In many ways, the emotional challenges of lymphedema mirror the physical challenges:

- Living well with the emotional and physical challenges of lymphedema are ongoing processes. Cancer may be cured or go into remission, but lymphedema is a chronic condition that must be managed for life.

- Lymphedema develops during periods of emotional and physical vulnerability:

    - Primary lymphedema can appear at any time, although it is most likely to appear at birth or during adolescence.

    - Secondary lymphedema develops following illness and medical treatment, injury, or as a result of other physical issues.

- Lymphedema, and associated emotional issues, may suddenly act up in response to something in the environment or for no apparent reason.

- Professional treatment can be helpful in dealing with emotional and physical symptoms, although the types of therapy are very different.

- Ongoing self-management is essential for maintaining both emotional and physical health.

- Either the emotional or the physical aspects of lymphedema can be disabling, especially if they are not treated.

Dr. McMahon brings a unique perspective to this task:

- She is a thorough and well organized writer with a conversational writing style that is clear and easy-to-read.

- Her experience as a therapist helps her understand real world issues and the most effective ways to help people change their thinking and actions.

- She believes passionately in empirically validated treatments and helps develop the best practice standards for the HMO where she works.

Dr. McMahon's book will help you understand the emotional challenges of lymphedema and, if necessary, change your thinking and behavior to overcome them. Her advice is valuable for anyone with lymphedema, or other chronic medical conditions, as well as friends and family, medical professionals, and psychotherapists.

This book serves as an ongoing reference as life situations, and the emotional challenges of lymphedema, change over time. The comprehensive nature of this book makes it possible to continue learning as you face different emotional challenges. This is not a book to be read once and tucked away; it is a resource and tool set that you can continue to use as you live well with lymphedema.

Ann Ehrlich

Acknowledgements

First, I want to thank you—the reader—for taking the time to read and consider the ideas presented here. This book is for you.

I also want to thank my patients. Your courage in successfully confronting and skillfully coping with physical and emotional difficulties is inspiring. It is an honor to work with you. Your successes fill me with respect and hope.

Thanks to my extended family. You are models for successfully overcoming life's challenges and creating lives of meaning, worth, and joy.

Thank you, always, to my husband and my daughter. Your unfailing love and support mean more to me than words can express.

Finally, thank you to each of the reviewers who gave generously of their time and expertise to make this book more accessible, helpful, and accurate:

Judith Fabian, PhD, ABPP

Fred Hirshberg, PhD

Laurie Katz, PhD

Claudia Kelsey

Karen Kohr-Blinn

Adrienne Lacavaro

Doris Laing, LMBT, CLT-LANA

Marilyn Lindsey, PhD

Ann Myers, MD

Harry Noda, PhD

Bonnie Pike

Barbara Pilvin

Ginny Pona

Carol Poole

M. Elise Radina, PhD

Sheila Ridner, PhD, RN

Pat Speckman

Saskia Thiadens, RN

Christine Thomas, MSPT, CLT-LANA

Alma Vinjé-Harrewijn, PT, CLT

Table of Contents

Contents in Brief

Contents in Detail

Lymphedema Isn't Just Physical

> **❝** Nobody talks about lymphedema! And even if they do, they focus on the physical aspects. Well, I have news for you! I have feelings too, as well as a body, and my feelings about lymphedema are a BIG issue.
> How come no one talks about this aspect of it? **❞**
> —*a frustrated lymphedema patient*!

Lymphedema impacts you emotionally as well as physically. This book will help you overcome the emotional challenges of lymphedema so you can adapt and thrive.

The book is designed to be a comprehensive, hands-on, practical guide. Feel free to use it the same way you would use a cookbook or a first aid manual. Those books cover everything from simple, normal everyday basics, like scrambling an egg or removing a splinter, to complicated tasks like creating a gourmet six-course meal or coping with a severe life-threatening emergency. Everything you might need to know is included.

This book takes a similar approach to the emotional challenges that accompany lymphedema. It covers the entire range of experience - from the normal, mild or temporary emotional reactions that most people experience, through the severe, disruptive problematic reactions that are less common. Everything you may need is included here.

Some parts of this book will apply to you immediately; some will not. You don't have to read every page. Feel free to skip around. Use what is relevant. The book is organized to help you find what you need, when you need it.

Worksheets are included throughout so you can track your progress and success. Turn to relevant chapters when new challenges arise or when old challenges rear their ugly heads again.

Life with lymphedema has its ups and downs emotionally, just like it does physically. Different sections will be more or less relevant to you at different times in your life with lymphedema.

Who This Book Is For (on page 3) below gives suggestions on how to find what will be most useful to you personally. Feel free to find and use those tips and tools that match your personal challenges.

This book was written for you. If you are hurting emotionally, it will give you tools and hope. If you are coping well with the emotional challenges of lymphedema, it provides tools to help you maintain your success over time.

When you read about reactions that you currently experience, I hope you will feel validated and encouraged. Other people have faced these challenges successfully and overcome them. You can, too.

When you read about challenges that do not reflect your present experience, I hope you will feel proud of your successful coping and grateful for struggles you do not face. You can skip those parts. Or you may want to read them in order to help others.

Why This Book Was Written

This book was born out of both my professional and my personal experience. Professionally, I see a lot of people with chronic medical problems because I work in a medical center as a clinical psychologist. My patients' courage and successes inspire me. Finding ideas or tools that help them is a tremendous joy. This book teaches you the tools that have been most helpful to my patients. Having a chronic illness myself, I can also assure you that I use many of these tools and personally find them helpful.

My specific personal interest in lymphedema began when a close relative developed it. We spoke at length. I researched the scientific literature. When I was invited to contribute the chapter on the emotional challenges of lymphedema for **Living Well With Lymphedema**, I realized how little was written on this area and how great the need is.

Other books on lymphedema focus primarily on dealing with the physical effects of lymphedema. (See Appendix A for a summary of the types of lymphedema, causes of lymphedema, complications of lymphedema and lymphedema treatment.) But the physical challenges of lymphedema are only part of the total picture.

Lymphedema is a chronic, fluctuating condition. It can be hard for doctors to diagnose. Treatment is time-consuming, costly, and sometimes uncomfortable. Dealing with lymphedema day after day can be demanding and frustrating, both physically and emotionally!

Negative emotional reactions are perfectly natural; yet, if these understandable reactions are not handled well, they can damage relationships, undermine commitment to necessary self-care, or decrease your quality of life. Living well with lymphedema means coping with the emotional challenges of lymphedema as well as the physical ones.

You have the ability to overcome these challenges. You can enjoy a happier and healthier life. You can create an enjoyable life full of satisfactions. You can thrive emotionally. My wish for you is that this book gives you all the knowledge and tools you may need to achieve your goals.

Who This Book Is For

This book is for people with lymphedema, their friends and family, parents of children with lymphedema, medical professionals, and psychotherapists. There are different benefits and reading paths for each group.

People with lymphedema

If you have lymphedema and would like to:

- Cope more skillfully and successfully with the challenges you face.

- Improve your communication and relationships with friends, family, and healthcare professionals.

- Live a happier, more satisfying life despite lymphedema.

- Sustain your gains over time.

I recommend that you read, and work through, Sections I through V. If you feel you are already coping well emotionally and primarily wish to protect and maintain this over time, I recommend that you read Chapter 5 and Section V.

Friends and family

If you have a friend or family member with lymphedema and would like to:

- Better understand their experience.

- Learn communication skills that can strengthen your relationship.

- Support them in overcoming the emotional challenges of lymphedema.

- Deal skillfully with your own emotional challenges.

I recommend that you read Chapter 22 first, and then read as much of Sections I through V and Appendix A as you need.

Parents of a child with lymphedema

If you are parenting a child with lymphedema and would like to:

- Better understand your child's experience.

- Deal more skillfully with the emotions you experience as the parent of a child with a chronic illness.

- Adapt your parenting skills to meet your child's needs.

I recommend that you read Chapter 23 first, and then read as much of Sections I through V and Appendix A as you need.

Medical professionals

If you are a healthcare provider working with lymphedema patients and would like to:

- Better understand your patients' experience and emotions.

- Improve your communications and relationship with your patients.

- Increase patient satisfaction.

- Provide more effective care.

I recommend that you read Chapter 24 first, and then read as much of Sections I through V and Appendix A as you need.

Psychotherapists

If you provide psychotherapy to clients with lymphedema and would like to:

- Better understand your patients' experience and emotions.

- Increase patient satisfaction.

- Provide more effective and patient-centered care.

I recommend that you read Chapter 25 first and then read as much of Sections I through V and Appendix A as you need.

What You Will Gain

Reading this book and applying the skills you'll learn will help you:

- Understand and cope with the normal, predictable challenges of lymphedema

- Avoid common pitfalls in overcoming these challenges

- Recognize when normal reactions become problematic or destructive, and know where to go for further knowledge or help

- Deal more effectively and confidently with others, including family, friends, coworkers, strangers, and healthcare professionals

- Set and prioritize your goals

- Identify where you are in the process of changing to achieve your goals

- Choose specific, effective actions to reach your personal goals

- Improve interactions with others using specific communication skills

- Know the ten signs of good coping and six warning signs of ineffective coping

- Monitor your progress

- Maintain your gains

Benefits of Overcoming These Emotional Challenges

Overcoming the emotional challenges of lymphedema leads to:

- Improved self-image and self-confidence
- More happiness and pleasure in life
- Less emotional distress
- Better control of lymphedema's physical symptoms
- More satisfying relationships
- Increased quality of life

Chapter 1

It All Fits Together

If you have lymphedema, you have emotional reactions to handle as well as physical reactions because lymphedema causes both. How you do physically affects you emotionally—and vice versa.

Your physical symptoms, your actions, your thoughts, and your emotions *all affect each other*. Because they all interact, change in one area will help the others.

You have the power to make positive changes. This is the message of hope and empowerment throughout this book.

Bad News and Good News

First the bad news: lymphedema causes visible, physical symptoms because the accumulation of lymphatic fluid results in swelling (see Appendix A for details). It is a chronic condition, so it will not go away on its own. It requires both professional treatment and personal self-management. If you don't treat it effectively, it will worsen. Currently, there is no cure.

If untreated, lymphedema can cause a body part to swell to several times its normal size and can make it very heavy. It can cause pain, tissue damage, the loss of mobility, and life-threatening infections. Lymphedema can make it hard to wear normal clothes or do normal activities.

Now the good news: early, effective, and consistent treatment reduces swelling. Self-management helps control symptoms, prevent or minimize flare-ups, and prevent deterioration. You can affect the course and severity of your lymphedema.

How you handle lymphedema, emotionally and physically, has a powerful impact. Emotional health makes physical health and functioning more likely.[1] You can strengthen your emotional health.

You are not helpless. You can make a difference. This book will give you the tools.

How It Fits Together

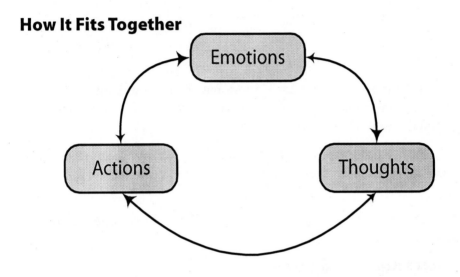

Figure 1-1: How It All Fits Together

We are feeling, thinking, and acting human beings.

- **Emotions** influence thoughts because you are more likely to have thoughts that fit how you feel at that moment.

  - Here's a positive example. When you feel confident or happy, you are more likely to remember successes or have spontaneous thoughts like, "*I can do this!*"

- **Thoughts** trigger emotions because your feelings about things are influenced by what you think about what is happening. In other words, your expectations, interpretations, and conclusions affect how you react.

  - Here's another positive example. Thoughts like, "*I can't make lymphedema go away, but I can do things to control it. I'm going to make my life the best it can be,*" help you feel more determined, upbeat, and good about yourself.

- **Actions** are guided by both emotions and thoughts. And in turn, your actions affect your thoughts, your emotions and, most importantly, your body – and your lymphedema.

  - Here's a negative example. If you feel discouraged, and you think, *"It's no use even trying self-management. I know I'll fail,"* you are likely to not use bandages, compression garments, or self-massage. As a result, your swelling may increase; you feel more hopeless; and you have more thoughts about being a *"loser and a failure."*

As the examples above show, the cycle of interaction among emotions, thoughts, and actions can be negative—or positive. You will learn how to make it positive.

The Impact of Your Emotions

Let's first explore in more detail some examples of the impact of your emotions. Caring for yourself emotionally. Feelings affect:

- **Thoughts:** For example, when you feel sad, angry, discouraged, frightened or self-conscious, you are more likely to have negative and upsetting thoughts enter your mind.

- **Actions:** If you feel depressed, hopeless, or overwhelmed, you are less likely to take care of yourself physically.

The Impact of Your Thoughts

Now let's focus on the impact of your thoughts. Thoughts affect:

- **Emotions:** What you find your mind automatically dwelling on, and what you deliberately choose to think about, both affect your emotional state. If you tell yourself that you're stupid, repulsive, or hopeless, you won't feel hopeful, encouraged, and confident. Dwelling on negatives makes you feel bad. Dwelling on positives and on what you can do makes you feel better.

- **Actions:** You take action based on what you believe is true and what you think is appropriate. If you think that things are hopeless or overwhelming, you won't try. If you think that you have a good chance of success, you will try.

The Impact of Your Actions

Finally, let's think about the impact of your actions. Actions affect:

- Emotions: What you do influences which emotions you feel, how severe they become, how long they last, and how much they disrupt your life. You can deliberately engage in actions designed to change your emotions. Specific examples are given throughout the book.

- Thoughts: You can deliberately engage in actions designed to change your thoughts. For example, talking or writing about something can change how you think about it. Trying new actions results in new knowledge, increased skill, and more success. New information, improved skills, and experiencing success can change your thoughts about the situation, about your options, and about yourself.

- Body: Actions, such as self-massage and self-management, directly affect the severity of your lymphedema symptoms and your risk of complications.

What's the bottom line? *Dealing well with your emotions helps you live well with lymphedema.*

How It All Fits Together in Your Life

This is a hands-on book and the worksheets are here for you to use. The more you interact with the book, the more benefit you will get from it. In fact, I hope that reading this book will be like having an ongoing conversation with pauses for reflection and skill-building.

Think about how your emotions, thoughts, and actions all interact. Use **Worksheet 1-1: How It All Fits Together in My Life** on page 13 to see how these factors fit together for you in positive and/or negative ways:

- Write down your specific lymphedema-related body sensations in the first column. For example, lightness or heaviness, pain or comfort, etc.

- Think about the specific emotions that are triggered by each feeling and write them in the second column.

- Write the thoughts that accompany these emotions in the third column.

- Notice how these emotions and thoughts affect what you do (your actions) and write this in the fourth column.

An example of how you might use this worksheet is on page 12: After you have completed the worksheet, look for positive cycles you want to strengthen or negative cycles that you want to change.

The Emotional Impact of Lymphedema

❝ This is a chronic disease….I hate [it]….I'm having a harder time with this than I did with breast cancer. There's no life or death urgency, no drama, just a constant dull ache and this hideous-looking hand and arm. I need role models for how to handle this. Supreme Court justices and movie stars get breast cancer, first ladies, famous novelists, and rock stars, but no one gets lymphedema. Or admits to having it anyway….I feel grotesque and don't want to be touched.[2] **❞**

Being diagnosed with lymphedema is a life-altering event. Suddenly, your body doesn't function like it did before. It doesn't look or feel the same.

Your self-image and interactions with others may change. You can't do things like you used to. Activities you took for granted may now be difficult – or even dangerous.

Lymphedema has moved into your life uninvited and unwanted – and it's not going to leave. Naturally, you have emotional reactions to this state of affairs.

At times, you may find yourself blind sided by emotional reactions. You can even feel as if you've been dropped into the middle of a minefield – without a map. The purpose of this book is to help you navigate this emotional minefield safely and effectively.

What to Expect

You want to know what to expect as a result of having lymphedema. In particular, you want to know when what you're feeling is a **normal and predictable** emotional reaction.

Example of Worksheet 1-1: How It All Fits Together

Body Sensations	Emotional Reactions	Thoughts	Actions
Swollen arm	Hopelessness, Anger, Sorrow, Fear, Resignation, Determination	"I'll never look like my old self again. I can't wear my wedding ring. What if this gets worse and worse? I need to contact my lymphedema therapist. We'll deal with this."	Cry. Call a supportive friend. Read about self-care. Go to a support group or find support and information online. Increase self-care. Check with lymphedema therapist.

This knowledge is reassuring and comforting because it helps you realize that:

- You are not alone.

- You are not crazy.

- You are not weak.

- You don't have to criticize yourself for having natural emotional responses.

- You don't have to beat yourself up about feeling bad.

- You don't have to worry on top of feeling distressed.

- Normal emotional reactions fluctuate and so you may feel sad, angry, scared, accepting, hopeful, happy, and so on from day to day, or even at different times in a single day.

- Distress can lessen with time, knowledge, and use of the coping skills in this book.

Worksheet 1-1: How It All Fits Together in My Life

Body Sensations	Emotional Reactions	Thoughts	Actions

Normal Reactions: An Overview

When you are diagnosed with lymphedema, you may feel confused, sad, angry, and scared. You may feel trapped, helpless, hopeless, or betrayed. You may grapple with questions of why this happened to you. It may stir up old emotions from the past and it certainly can make you feel stressed in the present.

These are normal reactions.

The bad news is that these common, normal reactions are distressing. They can strain your relationships with other people or make it harder for you to do what is needed to manage your lymphedema.

The good news is that the more you know about what to expect, the less you will feel overwhelmed by your emotions. You can cope with these normal reactions.

Many of these emotions naturally lessen and change over time. It has been said that, on average, it takes a year to come to terms with a major life change like the onset of a chronic condition. The more skillfully you work with your emotions, the faster this process occurs.

At the same time, lymphedema is not a static condition. Just as physical symptoms can improve and then worsen, emotional reactions can flare up, too. The book is designed so that you can turn to whichever section you may need, whenever you may need it.

Problematic Reactions: An Overview

Sometimes your emotional reactions, while understandable, may be less common and more problematic than the more common, predictable emotional reactions to lymphedema. For example, a normal, expected feeling can change into a problematic response if, instead of improving, it spirals into a vicious cycle and keeps getting worse.

Let's talk a bit about what I mean by problematic reactions.

Problematic emotional reactions are more long lasting, more severe, and/or more pervasive than the common, normal reactions. They interfere with your functioning in some important way. For example, if your normal feeling of anger or sadness becomes so strong or so ever-present that you end all your relationships or you completely stop caring for your lymphedema even though it is getting worse, then natural reactions have become problematic.

Sometimes emotional reactions qualify as problematic not because they are particularly intense, but because they are a chronic, ongoing burden that eats away at you over time, undermining your happiness and your capacities.

You do not have to be the victim of such emotional reactions.

I did *not* choose to cover the more troublesome "problematic" emotional reactions because I believe everyone with lymphedema experiences them. Indeed, I wrote this book because I have faith in your ability to handle lymphedema successfully and well.

I *did* choose to cover them, along with the more common "normal" emotional challenges, because everyone is different and because, like most things, emotions are not all-or-nothing. They fall along a continuum. They fluctuate. You may very well have reactions at times that fall between the artificial extremes of normal and problematic.

You are a unique individual. Your individual response to lymphedema's difficulties will be influenced by your personality, your past experiences, and your present situation.

I want you to have the full range of tools available. My goal is for you to be able to successfully handle your emotional responses so your emotions support, rather than undermine, your ability to care for your lymphedema.

Twelve Predictable Emotional Reactions

Section II (Chapters 2-13) presents twelve emotional challenges that commonly accompany lymphedema. Each has its own chapter and each chapter follows a common format.

First, you learn about the normal, although challenging, emotional reaction. Then you learn about related problematic reactions and how to tell if this is an issue for you. Specific coping suggestions are found throughout each chapter and, at the end of each chapter, you have a list of additional resources.

I expect you can successfully handle the normal, predictable reactions on your own using the coping suggestions along with some of the more general skills taught throughout this book.

Problematic reactions may be more difficult to change. The skills will help, but be prepared to work harder and longer and to use more of the skills. Sometimes professional help is required to successfully overcome such responses.

Some of the common psychological terms for problematic patterns of emotions and actions are covered in this book. These terms are mentioned only because knowing them may help you find information that is relevant and helpful.

But here's the bottom line about psychological terminology: Don't get hung up on whether or not your experience would be given a specific name. What's important is recognizing if you have a problematic pattern—and learning ways to change it.

Powerful Tools That Work

Throughout the book, I offer you specific tools and ideas that have been effective for many people.

Many of the skills taught in this book come from *cognitive-behavioral psychotherapy*. Cognitive-behavioral therapy (CBT) is one of the most research-tested and clinically-proven approaches to changing feelings. As the name indicates, you change your emotions by making changes in your cognitions (thoughts) and your actions (behavior).

By deliberately changing what you think and how you act, you can change problematic emotions and decrease their negative effect on your life.

Let me emphasize again that this is not just my personal theory or the latest pop-psych fad. CBT has been tested repeatedly and found to be helpful.

In addition to what is taught in this book, most chapters include a list of resources where you can find more information about specific topics.

You Make a Difference

For these tools to work, you must learn them, practice them, and apply them. You can expect that the tools and ideas in this book will:

- Help normal distressing reactions resolve more quickly and completely

- Reduce problematic emotional reactions and decrease their interference in your life

- Increase your coping, your functioning, and your happiness

- Provide you with valuable life skills

You have good reasons to be optimistic. You can look forward with well-founded hope as you use what you learn.

Making an active effort to change what you think and do speeds up positive change. You may have to work at it, but the work is worth doing. The more knowledge, skill, and practice you bring to feeling better, the more likely you are to succeed.

> **66** *I refused to let this disease get me down any longer and I learned to fight back. It's been a lot of hard work [but] . . . I have most of my life back!* **99**

Taking Charge: My Emotional Challenges Worksheet

The worksheet for My Emotional Challenges will help you evaluate the impact of each emotional challenge on your life and how well you are coping with each challenge. Several copies of this worksheet are included in different parts of this book.

As you read Chapters 2 through 13 you'll be instructed to update the worksheet in Chapter 14 (on page 201). When you get to Chapter 14, your ratings will help you decide what changes, if any, you want to make.

Instructions for the My Emotional Challenges Worksheet

Each of the twelve emotional challenges is listed in the worksheet with columns where you can rate their effect on your life. This rating has three parts:

1. **Severity**: how much of a problem is each emotional challenge? Rate each challenge on a scale of 0 to 10 where something that is not an issue for you would be a 0 and a challenge that was causing problems would be a 10.

2. **Coping**: how well are you coping with each emotional challenge? Rate your level of coping with each challenge on a scale of 0 to 10 where 0 is unable to cope or function and 10 is coping very well, thank you.

3. **Red Flag**: is this a red flag item for you? See below for a definition of red flags.

The right column is for Priority, we'll discuss that when we get to Chapter 14.

Throughout the book, you will occasionally see the words "**Red Flag**". These words identify a situation that is dangerous or a problem that may be an emergency. If you are facing a challenge that warrants a **Red Flag** notice, consider making it your highest priority.

The 0-10 scales used in this book are a shorthand way for you to note and compare how you are doing on each emotional challenge and to track your progress. You define what the numbers mean.

Your goal is to reach a point where you feel that you are coping well emotionally and that the emotional challenge is not causing you major distress or having a major impact on your life – as you define this for yourself. When you see your severity ratings declining and your coping ratings rising, you are probably doing something right.

In Section III: Taking Charge, you will use the Emotional Challenges worksheet to decide what area you want to work on first. In Section V you'll use it to track and maintain your changes.

Thoughts as You Begin

Some people feel discouraged if they identify several areas that they want to change. Actually, having several areas for improvement is good news. It means that your overall quality of life may improve dramatically as you apply your new skills.

Remember:

• You only need to take one step at a time.

• Each positive change can make the next one easier.

• You don't have to tackle everything at once.

Worksheet 1-2: My Emotional Challenges

Emotional Challenge	Severity Rating 0 – 10	Coping Rating 0 – 10	Red Flag? Y/N	My Priorities
Feeling overwhelmed				
Sadness and grieving				
Anger and resentment				
Fear				
Self-protection				
Worry				
Increased body focus				
Self-consciousness				
Others' reactions				
Searching for meaning				
Trauma and core beliefs				
Current stress				

Notes

1   "Mental Illness and/or Mental health? Investigating Axioms of the Complete State Model of Health" by C. L. M. Keyes. *Journal of Consulting and Clinical Psychology*, 2005; 73(3):539-548.

2   **Writing Out The Storm: Reading and Writing Your Way Through Serious Illness or Injury** by Barbara Abercrombie. St. Martin's Griffin, 2002. pp. 125-126

The Emotional Challenges of Lymphedema

This section covers twelve emotional challenges commonly faced by people with lymphedema:

- Feeling overwhelmed
- Sadness and grieving
- Anger
- Fear
- Being self-protective
- Uncertainty and worry

- Focusing on your body
- Self-consciousness
- Handling others' reactions
- Asking "why?"
- Lessons from your past
- Current life stresses

The headings above include such issues as helplessness, feelings of loss, hopelessness, feeling abandoned by the medical profession, claustrophobia from garments or bandaging, uncertainty, self-isolation or withdrawal from others, loneliness, and feelings of shame or guilt.

For each emotional challenge, a range of normal responses is presented followed by a description of more severe reactions with checklists to help you decide whether this may be an issue for you personally. Specific suggestions for overcoming the challenge are found throughout each chapter. Each chapter ends with a list of additional resources for further information.

Chapter 2

Feeling Overwhelmed

You may never even have heard of lymphedema before you were diagnosed with it. You wonder what to do. You may feel alone

It can be hard to find useful information. The people you ask for guidance may not have answers. Or, even worse, they may be unhelpful or misinformed.

66 I felt so incredibly alone. I had never met anyone else with this condition. When I finally found a support group, I felt better already just knowing that there were other people out there who experienced the same things I go through. **99**

Normal: Feeling Overwhelmed, Then Coping

It is a perfectly normal reaction to be temporarily overwhelmed. It is certainly normal to have thoughts such as *"This is too much to deal with," "I want someone to take care of me," "I want this to just go away,"* or *"I want to run away."* These are understandable responses to finding yourself in a situation you didn't choose.

Because feeling uncertain or overwhelmed is uncomfortable, people respond by doing things designed to reduce the unpleasant feeling. Ideal responses are actively seeking information and finding ways to take charge.

You are taking this approach by reading this book. Take a moment, stop, and pat yourself on the back. Give yourself credit for tackling this problem head-on.

It is can be hard to rise to a challenge like lymphedema where there are many unknowns. Lymphedema may worsen at times without your knowing why. You may sometimes feel helpless, incompetent, or out of control.

You may be tempted to take a passive approach to the whole problem by giving up or avoiding thinking about it. The disadvantage of such a passive approach is that it is likely to fail because lymphedema that is not cared for worsens and can lead to complications.

It will not disappear if you procrastinate long enough. It will not improve if you avoid thinking about it. It will not go away if you don't pay attention to it.

Turning to sleep, distractions, fantasy, denial, passivity, overeating, alcohol, or drugs *as a substitute for successful coping* only creates additional problems.

Nancy Brinker reminisces in **Winning The Race:**[1]

> 66   The one problem I had not anticipated was lymphedema."
> When she was told by her physician that the swelling was irreversible, "I didn't accept that, and I don't think any woman   99
> should.

It took her a year, but she got her lymphedema controlled.

Always remember that lymphedema that is cared for can improve. Find safe, healthy ways to help yourself feel less overwhelmed by starting with the list of coping suggestions on page 25.

Problematic Passivity or Avoidance

How do you know if your response of feeling overwhelmed is moving from the temporary, predictable reaction into a more severe reaction that is likely to cause difficulties? Ask yourself these questions:

☐ Am I refusing to believe or accept that I have lymphedema?

☐ Am I kidding myself by thinking lymphedema will "go away by itself"?

☐ Do I completely avoid thinking about my lymphedema?

☐ Do I ask no questions and learn nothing about the condition?

☐ Do I pretend it doesn't exist and do nothing to improve it?

☐ Am I avoiding medical appointments or therapy sessions?

Coping Suggestions:

Find the information you need. The more you know what to do, the less overwhelmed you can feel.

Find people who support you emotionally and help you cope.

Give yourself mini-vacations from lymphedema. Let yourself periodically take "a break from lymphedema." Here are some examples:

☐ Immerse yourself in pleasurable activities or distraction.

☐ Escape temporarily through meditation or an appropriate amount of sleep.

☐ Turn to someone or something that comforts you, such as a person, a pet, or even a stuffed animal.

☐ If possible, arrange to briefly relinquish the burden of self-care by letting others care for you.

☐ Talk to your lymphedema therapist about when and how you can modify your self-care activities. Maybe there will be times when you can safely do less.

Temporary, deliberate, breaks help you return to the task of coping.

☐ Do I say things like "There's not enough time" or "It's too hard" to participate in treatment?

☐ Am I not following self-care recommendations?

☐ Am I engaging in risky behaviors or ignoring lymphedema precautions?

☐ Am I running away from this challenge by oversleeping, overeating, overspending, abusing drugs or alcohol, or other avoidance actions?

Pause for a moment and reflect on your answers. Are you running away, giving up, or passively waiting for someone to fix you?

- **If you think you are being passive or avoiding because of hopelessness,** read Chapter 3.

- **If you think you are acting this way because of your fears, worries, or self-consciousness,** read Chapters 5, 7, and 9 that deal with those emotions.

- **If you are using drugs or alcohol to avoid dealing with lymphedema,** read the information on chemical substances later in this chapter.

- **If you feel helpless or incompetent because of specific past experiences,** you may want to read Chapter 12.

Why Passivity and Avoidance Are Barriers to Overcoming

Giving up can be so tempting. Modern life makes distractions easy and seductive. The television is always there. The bed is always there. So is the refrigerator. There are computer games, chat rooms, books, and videos. Why not escape? Why not passively wait to feel better or for the problem to go away?

Well, one big reason these responses are problematic is that it is *your* body that has lymphedema. Only you can feel the early warning signs of worsening. Only you can learn what your body needs to improve. You are, unless you are paralyzed, the only person who can move your body in ways that help the lymph flow.

Your body is already doing the best it can. It needs your help.

Lymphedema therapists can help during treatments but your body has lymphedema 24 hours a day and you are the only person who is with your body 24 hours a day.

Your body needs you. Your body relies on you. Like a helpless child or a fragile flower, your body depends upon you for the care it needs to survive and flourish.

In reading this book, you are seeking ways to care both for your body and for your emotions. You are looking for a healthy balance in your life. Sometimes medicines or other chemicals can help you find such a balance.

The Role of Chemical Substances

People turn to chemical substances for all kinds of reasons. They use substances to: increase energy or calm down, be more alert or go to sleep, escape bad moods or increase good moods, stop pain or heighten sensations. Substances can include alcohol (beer, wine, or liquor), legal medicines and drugs (like sleeping pills, anti-anxiety medicines, pain pills, nicotine) and illegal drugs.

Substances can be helpful and increase your coping or they can be harmful and be used to help you avoid. How can you tell which is which?

Active Coping or Passive Avoidance?

A signal that substances are helpful and support active coping is that your self-care, your self-esteem, and/or your relationships improve as a result of using them. For example, pain medication may let you move around more and function better - helping you physically and emotionally. Antidepressants can lessen depression and anxiety - improving your thinking and functioning.

To help weigh the positive results against the negative results, ask yourself questions such as:

• Is my mood improved or worsened – either immediately or over time?

• Are my thinking and judgment improved or worsened?

• Does it harm my body?

A warning sign that substances are being used to avoid is when you use them to numb your feelings and to escape, rather than to cope and to overcome problems and difficult feelings.

Drugs, legal or illegal, can offer a tempting escape if you feel overwhelmed by lymphedema. Unfortunately, many are easy to abuse and can be physically or emotionally addicting.

If you notice **any** of the following, you may be abusing a substance:

☐ Because of substance use, you don't take care of your lymphedema or handle other responsibilities at home or work the way you know you should.

☐ The effects of substance use interfere with work or school or get you into legal trouble.

☐ You keep using even when it is dangerous or it hurts your relationships.

☐ In order to get your substance, you steal or use money that should be spent on lymphedema treatment and supplies.

If you have noticed **any** of the above, you may feel a lot better physically and emotionally if you decrease your use.

Successfully Overcoming Feeling Overwhelmed

Lymphedema can be hard. Think about how you support and guide yourself through the difficult times.

When you feel overwhelmed, find healthy ways to escape temporarily from lymphedema. Find ways to escape that strengthen and refresh you. Reread the "Coping Suggestions" earlier in this chapter for more ideas.

The signs of an effective escape are:

• The way you escape does not itself cause problems **and**

• You cope well when you return to the problem.

The signs of an ineffective escape are:

• The way in which you escape creates more problems.

• You *routinely* respond to feeling overwhelmed with passivity or avoidance.

• You feel weaker instead of stronger when you return to the problem.

You don't have the choice of not having lymphedema. You do choose how you respond to having it.

In life, the fewer choices we have, the more important it is that we make the best possible choices. The sooner and more actively you treat the lymphedema, the better your results can be.

Coping Suggestions:

Start small. Focus on what you can do.

Track your progress. Stretch yourself by doing a little more each week.

Learn what helps your body and improves your emotions. You will become more skilled, more knowledgeable, and more effective.

Fight back by supporting legislation to improve insurance coverage for lymphedema treatment, finding ways to support lymphedema research, helping others, spreading the word about lymphedema, or in other ways.

Join activities, such as a support group, swim class, lymphedema exercise class, or walking group, where you meet others who are successfully and actively coping with lymphedema.

Don't give up! Persevere. No matter what!

As Winston Churchill said, *"Never give in. Never, never, never, never…."* [2]

"   I live a normal life despite having lymphedema.
I refused to let this disease take over and instead I decided that **"**
I would take control of it!

As your body benefits from your actions, you will develop more confidence and pleasure in caring for it and helping it. As you actively face problems, you develop coping skills and solutions for which you can take credit.

You can feel real pride and deep satisfaction in caring for your body. Your efforts can result in improvement in your body and increase in positive emotions.

Feeling Overwhelmed and Its Impact on Your Life

Turn to Worksheet 14-2: **My Emotional Challenges** on page 201 and complete the line for "Feeling overwhelmed."

Resources

For changing a passive or avoidant approach to problems:

Successful Problem-Solving: A Workbook to Overcome the Four Core Beliefs That Keep You Stuck by Matthew McKay, PhD and Patrick Fanning. New Harbinger Publications, 2002.

For alcohol or substance abuse:

National Institute on Alcohol Abuse and Alcoholism (NIAAA) (www.niaaa.nih.gov)

Alcoholics Anonymous (AA) (www.aa.org)

Al-Anon and Ala-Teen (www.al-anon.alateen.org)

Secular Organizations for Sobriety (www.cfiwest.org/sos)

SMART Recovery Self-Help Network (Self-Management and Recovery Training) (www.smartrecovery.org)

Chemically Dependent Anonymous (www.cdaweb.org)

Adult Children of Alcoholics (www.AdultChildren.org)

Narcotics Anonymous (NA) (www.na.org)

Notes

1   **Winning the Race** by Nancy Brinker with Chriss Winston. Tapestry Press, 2001. p. 63.

2   Sir Winston Churchill 1874-1965. Speech, 1941, Harrow School – quote found on www.quotationspage.com

Chapter 3

Sadness and Grieving

Being sad after learning you have lymphedema is completely normal, especially if you've just been through treatment for cancer or an injury. It's a common reaction to feel, *"I got over the cancer – and now this!"*

You may feel disheartened. You may feel isolated and alone. You may be embarrassed to find yourself unexpectedly in tears at times. It has been said that it takes up to a year to adjust after being diagnosed with a serious illness or chronic condition.

Feelings of sadness and grief can occur or reoccur at any time. These feelings may have obvious triggers, like the anniversary of your diagnosis, or they may seem to just pop up out of the blue, for example in response to a song or a chance comment.

Normal Sadness and Grieving

What emotional reactions associated with sadness might you expect to feel as a normal response? You may find that you:

- Cry more easily.

- Alternate feeling numb, feeling sad, and feeling angry.

- Feel a sense of loss.

- Find it harder to enjoy things.

- Withdraw physically, socially, or emotionally as you grapple with the diagnosis and what it means.

• Feel alone and lonely.

These are understandable, normal reactions. When things change against your will, grieving is part of the process of adapting to the new situation. This is part of the human condition.

At the same time, acute grief is not meant to last forever. You should not become so trapped in sadness that you are unable to find any enjoyment in other aspects of life.

If you are experiencing a normal level of sorrow and grieving, your reactions will fluctuate, but every week that passes will gradually bring you closer to feeling better. This is especially true if you use the time wisely.

Coping Suggestions:

Acknowledge your painful emotions.

Actively come to terms with the changes in your body and your life.

Permit yourself to grieve the losses you are facing. Experience the feelings.

Grieving Your Losses

Lymphedema can be controlled and life can be good again, but learning that you have lymphedema does mean facing certain losses.

One big loss is the luxury of taking your body for granted and of being unthinking in your treatment of your body. The way your body looks and functions is now affected by lymphedema and you need to actively help your body move the lymph.

When your body no longer handles an essential task automatically, and you must shoulder the responsibility, this is a loss of your freedom to be un-thinking. This adds tasks to your daily responsibilities that people without lymphedema don't have and are unlikely to understand.

Is your lymphedema the result of an illness or accident? If so, the lymph-edema diagnosis may bring back some of the grief you felt as a result of the original illness or accident.

Sally's Story

I have found that dealing with the lymphedema is more difficult than dealing with my breast cancer. Perhaps it is the constant reminder of all I have lost. I was extremely physically fit and strong. I maintained a huge garden and a small orchard which I no longer have the strength to do. I can't pick up my children or carry my own groceries. Bandaging takes time.

The exact losses and their importance vary from person to person:

- You may feel you have lost your attractiveness, your ability to wear attractive fashionable clothes, or your hopes for the future.

- You may feel a loss of independence, health, or freedom.

- You may lose, or have to modify, activities you enjoyed such as steamy hot showers, long soaking hot baths, or gardening with your bare hands.

- Dealing with hot weather, traveling by plane, and other activities now present challenges that have to be taken into account and planned for in advance.

- You may feel as if there is an invisible wall restricting you and shutting you off from the world you used to inhabit and that others still enjoy.

- If you have primary lymphedema, your children may inherit this condition.

Circle any of the losses listed above that are true for you. Think about any other losses that are personally important to you. This helps you identify what you need to grieve. It will also help you track your progress through grief to acceptance and moving forward.

Moving from Grieving to Acceptance

In Worksheet 3-1: **Moving from Grieving to Acceptance** on page 35, list what you have lost because of lymphedema. You may have already come to terms with these losses or you may be actively grieving them now. Of course, feelings of grief and sadness may vary from day to day depending on what happens in your life. For this worksheet, think about how you are generally doing overall.

For each loss, reflect and rate where you are now on the path to acceptance using a scale of 0 to 10 where 0 is no acceptance or intense grief and 10 is full acceptance or at peace. What the numbers mean varies from person to person. Use them to help *you* evaluate where you are now and to track your progress. For example, you might give yourself a score of 0 if every day you feel all-consuming, intense grief and have no acceptance at all.

Reaching full acceptance and peace (a score of 10 on all losses) is probably an unrealistic goal; but as you move in that direction, you should notice a marked increase in your happiness and quality of life. The energy you used for grieving will have been freed for enjoying life's pleasures and mastering life's challenges. Instead of looking backward, you will be focusing on the present and planning for the future.

Coping Suggestions:

Remind yourself that the purpose of grieving is to lead to acceptance.

Grieve. Then turn to living the best life you can. As you do this, the pain of loss and mourning becomes less. Acceptance grows. Feelings of depression lessen. More and more, you focus on what remains and what you can do. This is the progression you want to see.

Ask yourself whether you are seeing this progression from grief to acceptance. If you are, notice what helps you resolve your grief. If you are not, notice what thoughts and actions you keep repeating as you remain stuck.

Talk to people who care and who make you feel better.

Do things that bring you pleasure or that give you a sense of accomplishment.

Worksheet 3-1: Moving from Grieving to Acceptance

My Level of Acceptance (0-10)										
My Losses										

You can become trapped in feelings of sorrow, grief, negativity, or hopelessness. When this happens, your normal reaction of temporary sadness and grieving does not resolve. Temporary depression may turn into clinical depression.

Problematic Sadness and Grieving: Depression

The words "depressed" and "depression" have entered everyday language. As a result, it can be hard to know what people really mean when they talk about depression. In this book, I will try to use the word "depression" as it is defined by psychologists and psychiatrists.

Two Types of Depression

Two common patterns of depression are:

- **Major depression**, which is a depression that is characterized by its severity and

- **Dysthymia**, which is milder but long-lasting.

Major Depression

Your thinking changes and narrows in a major depression. It focuses on the negative. You view the world through a dark, negative filter. Bad memories come easily; optimistic thinking seems like self-delusion. The future can seem hopeless and bleak. You may blame or despise yourself or see yourself as unloved, unworthy, helpless, or a burden to others. You may withdraw from people. You may find yourself wanting to die.

Dawn's Story

Since the diagnosis, I can't seem to move on. Most days I just sit and stare at the TV. I don't care what's on. Sometimes I cry but mostly I'm just numb.

I can barely drag myself out of bed in the morning and I can barely drag myself back into bed at night, yet I don't sleep very well. I'm always tossing and turning. I don't eat much and I have no interest in doing anything, not even lymphedema self-care.

You may be having what is called a major depression, if, after a few weeks:

- You continue to feel sad, depressed, or empty for most of the time on most days or

- Activities that you would normally enjoy bring you little pleasure.

A major depression is even more likely if you also experience five or more of these changes on most days for two or more weeks:

☐ Change in weight and appetite (either a marked increase or decrease)

☐ Change in sleep (either more or less)

☐ Tiredness, waking not rested, loss of normal energy

☐ Trouble concentrating

☐ Being so agitated or slowed down that others see the difference in you

☐ Feeling worthless or guilty

☐ Thoughts of suicide or wanting to die

Dysthymia

Loss or stress is more likely to trigger a serious depression if you have had one or more episodes of depression in the past or if you have struggled with a condition known as dysthymia.

Dysthymia is like a low-grade chronic depression. People who struggle with dysthymia have milder symptoms that are present on most days for two or more years. This is different from having periods of depression that alternate with periods of extreme high energy.

Two or more of these signs are present on most days:

☐ Either poor sleep or appetite or chronic oversleeping or overeating

☐ Ongoing easy fatigue or low energy

☐ Ongoing trouble concentrating or making decisions

☐ Chronic low self-esteem

☐ Chronic hopelessness or negativity.

When Depression Is an Emergency

RED FLAG:

If you find yourself making plans to kill yourself, **treat this as an emergency and get help**.

Do not make permanent, life-or-death decisions while your thinking is distorted by depression.

Find immediate support and appropriate care. Call a local or national suicide hotline, or friends or family who help you feel better and get treatment.

Contact a mental health professional and/or your healthcare provider and start treatment for depression. See Chapter 19.

How Common Is Depression?

If you are feeling depressed, you are not alone. Depression is common.

It affects almost twice as many women as men and it is more common among older adults and cancer survivors. In the US, 12 percent of women and 6.6 percent of men are affected by a depressive disorder each year.[1]

An estimated 20% of older adults in the community, and as many as 50% in nursing homes, suffer from depression.[2] In one survey of cancer survivors 70% of respondents said they had to deal with depression as a result of their cancer and 88% of this group said they had some level of difficulty dealing with the issue.[3]

Temporary depression is a very normal response to a life stress like lymphedema. It is one of our body's coping mechanisms. Many people find that they have trouble focusing or sleeping as they come to grips with a new situation. Plus, of course, sleep can be more difficult due to physical symptoms of lymphedema, the weight or heat of garments or bandages, or pain from lymphedema or other causes.

The Bad News and Good News about Depression

The bad news: Staying depressed is not good for your mental or physical health. Depression can be self-perpetuating. It can feed on itself in a vicious cycle. Depression may be a familiar problem or it may be something that you have never before encountered.

Ongoing depression is associated with worse physical health and increased likelihood of death. Depression in older adults not only causes distress and suffering but also interferes with physical, mental, and social functioning. Older Americans have the highest suicide rate of any age group, and depression is the biggest risk factor for suicide.[4]

The good news: Deliberately changing your thinking and actions can help life depressed mood. Self-help skills from books (such as this one and the books listed below), activities, and social support can all help.

If self-help is not enough, there are many treatments available which have proven their effectiveness in well-designed research studies. Antidepressant medication (alone or with other medicines) is often combined with psycho-therapy and has proven effectiveness. Cognitive-behavioral and interpersonal psychotherapies, sometimes combined with medication, have proven effectiveness. Some people may find other psychotherapies helpful. For extremely severe, life-threatening, treatment-resistant depressions, electro-convulsive therapy can be a life-saving option. If you, or others who know you, see the signs of depression, get help.

Julie's Story

I thought I was coping well but after a while I realized that I had stopped smiling and laughing. Friends and loved ones asked me what was wrong. My world was grey, nothing was fun, and I often felt weepy.

My support group kept me going. With professional help, I was able to solve the practical problems and work through my feelings. I'm so glad I did because now I'm able to enjoy life again. The sun does shine. Jokes are funny. I'm not snapping at my family like I used to do and the future is something to look forward to with pleasure.

Sadness And Grieving: Their Impact On Your Life

Think about your answers to the questions and worksheets in this chapter. Review your answers and what you have learned.

Now, turn to Worksheet 14-2: **My Emotional Challenges** on page 201 and complete the line for "Sadness and grieving."

Resources

Authentic Happiness by Martin Seligman, PhD. Free Press, 2004.

Control Your Depression by Peter Lewisohn, PhD, Ricardo Munoz, PhD, Mary Ann Youngren, PhD, and Antonette Zeiss, PhD. Fireside, 1992.

Feeling Good: The New Mood Therapy by David Burns, MD. Avon, 1999.

The Feeling Good Handbook by David Burns, MD. Plume Books, 1999.

How to Stubbornly Refuse to Make Yourself Miserable about Anything – Yes, Anything! by Albert Ellis, PhD. Carol Publishing, 1988.

Learned Optimism: How to Change Your Mind and Your Life by Martin Seligman, PhD. Simon and Schuster, 1990.

Mind Over Mood: Change How You Feel by Changing the Way You Think by Dennis Greenberger, PhD and Christine Padesky, PhD. Guilford Publications, 1995.

Overcoming Depression: A Step-by-Step Approach to Gaining Control Over Depression, 2 ed. by Paul Gilbert. Oxford University Press, 2001.

Notes

1   Data from NIMH (www.nimh.nih.gov/publicat/womensoms.cfm) accessed on July 15, 2005. Data from Regier DA, Narrow WE, Rae DS, et al. The de facto mental and addictive disorders service system. Epidemiologic Catchment Area prospective 1-year prevalence rates of disorders and services. Archives of General Psychiatry, 1993; 50(2): 85-94.

2   Data from the American Psychological Association (www.apa.org/ppo/issues/olderdepressfact.html) accessed on July 15, 2005.

3   LIVESTRONG Poll Fact Sheet by the Lance Armstrong Foundation, November 30, 2004.

4   Data from the American Psychological Association (www.apa.org/ppo/issues/olderdepressfact.html) accessed on July 15, 2005.

Chapter 4

Anger

> **❝** I don't remember ever being so mad. Here I had suffered through the cancer, endured chemotherapy….and now this.[1] **❞**

Anger and resentment are natural emotional reactions to learning that you have lymphedema. Anger is part of the "fight-or-flight" response that is automatically triggered when you are confronted by a threat.

Resentment is a common form of simmering anger. It can be triggered by perceptions of loss, deprivation, injustice, etc.

Do not blame yourself for feeling anger or resentment. They are normal and you don't control your feelings. *However, you do control your actions.*

Normal Anger and Resentment

Anger and resentment may be directed at yourself or at others. You may be angry about present problems or past events. Your anger may have many targets and/or triggers.

Normal Anger Targets or Triggers

You may relive the anger you felt about the original cause of the lymphedema. If your secondary lymphedema is a result of surgery or cancer treatment, you may be furious with the doctors. If it is a result of burns or an accident, you may relive your rage at whomever you feel is responsible.

You may wonder *"Why me?"* and find yourself swept up in gusts of anger and resentment at other people who don't have to deal with this problem. Why are they healthy when you are not?

You may be angry with the entire medical profession. You may have thoughts such as *"They gave me this!" "They didn't warn me!" "Why isn't there a cure?" "Why isn't there more research?" "Why aren't there more treatment options?" "Why doesn't my doctor know more?" "Why aren't there answers to my questions about what to expect? "They don't listen!" "They just abandoned me."*

If you were not warned about the possibility of lymphedema or if you were not told how to protect yourself against lymphedema, you may feel betrayed by your healthcare team.

If you were taking preventive actions and got lymphedema anyway, it is natural to feel angry and think, *"I did what I was supposed to do and I still got lymphedema. It's just not fair!"* You may get angry at yourself. *"Why didn't I do more? I could have/should have prevented this."*

If you have primary lymphedema and it runs in the family, you may be angry with the parent from whom you inherited it. If no reason can be found, you may blame your parents, the medical profession, or want to lash out at fate. You may resent the fact that other people don't have the condition.

If you are the parent of a child with lymphedema, you may be angry with yourself, or at your spouse, for transmitting the condition. You may resent the demands on money and time. (See Chapters 11 and 23 for help with guilt and blame.)

It is also very natural to be angry if you have to struggle to find information and help. Your insurance may not cover the treatment you need. You may be angry at having to do more paperwork and make more appointments. You face a chronic health problem. You have to make changes in your daily life. Maybe you can't wear your shoes or clothes, your wedding ring or jewelry. Maybe no one warned you and you got sunburned through your compression garment.

The Purpose of Anger

Anger is a normal, natural, and healthy emotion. It is a signal that there is a problem. Its purpose is to energize and activate you so you take effective action to protect yourself and to fight the problem.

> ### *Coping Suggestions:*
>
> Admit that you are angry.
>
> Find safe ways to express your anger. You might write it out or talk it out. If your lymphedema permits, do physical tasks like walking out your anger or pounding on a pillow. Express it in your imagination or through drawing, music, or other means.
>
> Remind yourself that anger, in and of itself, is not bad. It is just a feeling and feelings are just feelings. Feelings come whether you want them or not. You don't choose what feelings spontaneously arise. You do, however, make important choices about what you do in response to your feelings.
>
> Focus on what you can change.

Transient anger that alerts you to problems and stimulates you to find solutions is helpful.

Anger Cautions

Please understand: I am not suggesting that you express your anger in words or actions without restraint. Nor am I recommending that you nurse resentment and stew in anger, no matter how real and justified your grievances may be. At the same time, I am not suggesting that you pretend to yourself that you are not angry or resentful when you are.

Blindly acting on your anger often results in more anger. Chronic, unresolved anger can destroy the quality of your life. Denying that you are angry keeps you from finding solutions.

Any of these three options can harm your relationships and your health.[2] Let's start by learning more about anger.

Two Common Misunderstandings about Anger

Two ideas about anger are widely believed to be true. The first is that people are not in control of their behavior when they are angry. The second is that anger has to be let out or else it will never go away.

Both statements are false. They reflect common misunderstandings about anger. Let's discuss these false beliefs because they can contribute to problematic anger.

False Belief 1: Anger is Uncontrollable

One common misconception about anger is that anger takes people over so that they *"can't control themselves"* when they are angry. This is not true.

There are only a very few situations in which a person could be considered "out of control" of their anger. One would be when the person is truly out of touch with reality because of a serious illness, such as psychosis, mania, or dementia. Another would be when the person's judgment, impulse control, or ability to think, are seriously impaired by alcohol or drugs.

You are in control of your actions, even when you are angry.

 RED FLAG:

If you think one of the examples above is true for you and that you are truly "out of control" of your actions, seek professional help immediately.

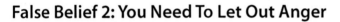

False Belief 2: You Need To Let Out Anger

The second common misunderstanding is that the only way to decrease anger is to *"let it out."* People used to believe that anger was like pressure inside and you needed let it out in words and actions. You may still hear people advising you to "let off steam". Only part of the thinking behind this suggestion is true.

Yes, you should acknowledge your feelings. Yes, accept that you have whatever feelings you have, even when they are uncomfortable to yourself or others. Yes, take action based on your anger. However, here's the important thing to understand. It is NOT automatically helpful to express angry thoughts and feelings.

Acting on your anger can be helpful, it can be useless, or it can be actively dangerous and destructive. Anger may lead you to educate others and advocate for changes in treatment. That can be helpful. Anger may cause you to throw your bandages across the room - perfectly understandable, but not very helpful. Anger may lead you to cancel appointments and recklessly defy treatment recommendations – actively harmful because it puts you at risk.

Simply expressing anger, while doing nothing to resolve or lessen it, sometimes only increases or sustains your anger.

This is very important, so let me repeat it, *Letting out your anger, without using your judgment and without identifying and resolving the underlying problem, only feeds your anger."*

Three Types of Problematic Anger

Problematic anger can take three forms: abusive anger, chronic anger, or denied anger. Let's look at each in turn starting with the least common but most serious.

Type 1: Abusive Anger

You let anger guide your actions regardless of the consequences. You lash out and are verbally or physically abusive.

This is like driving a car by closing your eyes while slamming your foot down on the accelerator. It is dangerous, hurtful, and causes physical or emotional damage.

Abusive anger channels the energy of your anger into destruction instead of harnessing it for problem solving. You may scream at others, call them names, and/or threaten to hurt them. You may destroy objects of value to yourself or others. You may act in ways that are dangerous.

 RED FLAG:

If you shove, push, slap, punch, hit, or choke others—or if you threaten them with weapons, this is physical abuse. **Treat it as an emergency** and immediately seek help through anger management training, psychotherapy, or medication.

Type 2: Chronic Anger, Hostility, and/or Cynicism

With chronic anger, you don't just feel angry briefly; you stay angry for long periods of time. You simmer. You may feel generally hostile toward others.

You cynically expect the worst. Low-grade anger becomes a constant in your life.

This is a bit like driving the car while pressing both the gas pedal and the brake. You don't impulsively crash into things, but it puts terrible stress on the engine. Chronic anger, hostility, or cynicism is harmful to your health.

Are you simmering with anger rather than boiling over? Ask yourself:

☐ Am I frequently irritable or short with friends, family, coworkers, or healthcare professionals?

☐ Do I often respond angrily, inwardly or outwardly, to the general annoyances of daily life or to the specific annoyances and demands of life with lymphedema?

☐ Do I find myself thinking over and over about others' mistreatment of me?

☐ Do I automatically attribute negative motives to others or repeatedly have thoughts like *"People are just out for what they can get," "They're deliberately doing this to upset me,"* or *"You've got to look out for Number One all the time because everyone else is."*

☐ Do I often feel attacked, demeaned, criticized, or let down by many people?

☐ Do I normally expect the worst from everyone I meet and believe that this is appropriate and justified?

If you answered yes to one or more of the above, you may be experiencing chronic anger.

What are the problems with this approach to life with lymphedema?

Chronic Anger Is Unhealthy

Research on heart disease originally thought that people who are always in a hurry, who are driven to get a lot done, and who are competitive or impatient, were at greater risk for heart disease. They were labeled "Type A" people.

Only one part of that was found to be correct. Additional research has shown that the most dangerous and damaging factor is a chronically hostile, angry, cynical approach to the world and other people. People with this attitude are more likely to get heart disease and other illnesses.[3]

Chronic Anger Can Be a Sign of Depression

When we are depressed, we are flooded with negative thoughts. If these negative thoughts make us feel hopeless and teary, we are likely to recognize this as depression.

However, when the negative thoughts make us irritable, hostile, or cynical, we may not realize that the underlying problem is depression. Depression interferes with caring for lymphedema.

Chronic Anger Harms Relationships

A hostile, cynical approach to life and to other people makes it very difficult to form and maintain mutually trusting, supportive relationships. Research studies have repeatedly shown that having supportive relationships is one of the main factors associated with good health, longer life, greater happiness, and better quality of life overall.

Type 3: Denied Anger

With denied anger, you refuse to admit to yourself and others that you are angry. Because the existence of anger is not acknowledged, neither the anger nor the underlying cause is ever resolved.

This is rather like refusing to do preventive maintenance on the car and ignoring warning signs unless the car breaks down completely. At worst, the car stops functioning and you have no idea why or what to do to fix it. At best, you lose valuable information vital to keeping your car performing smoothly, effectively, and in top condition over the long haul.

You may deny to yourself or to other people that you feel angry about lymphedema because you feel guilty or frightened about feeling angry. You may deny feeling resentment that others don't understand, don't help, or don't face the difficulties you face. You may decide that you cannot feel this way and that you must never admit it or express it.

Do not confuse feeling and thought with action. You are responsible for your actions. You are not responsible for the thoughts and feelings that spontaneously arise within your mind. You don't control these so you have nothing for which to feel guilty.

If you try to censor yourself so that you do not think or feel, you cut yourself off from what is going on inside emotionally. This prevents you from figuring out what other feelings may be behind the anger and it keeps you from noticing warning signs of underlying problems.

Anger that is never acknowledged stays inside. Unresolved, denied feelings do not go away. They can make it hard to feel positive feelings. They can interfere with relationships. Unresolved, denied feelings often go underground and affect your body. With lymphedema, you don't want your body stressed.

When you are not consciously aware of your emotions, you are more likely to experience physical symptoms, such as skin problems, unexplained aches and pains, or a general feeling of malaise. You may find yourself overeating to try to "stuff down" your anger.

Anger may make you and other people uncomfortable, but if you can't admit that you're angry, how can you resolve it and move on to more positive emotions? If anger triggers aren't examined, they don't get resolved and you lose valuable opportunities to grow in communication skills and to improve your life. You want anger triggers related to lymphedema resolved and you want close, supportive relationships to help you deal with lymphedema over time.

Anger Is a Signal

Anger is an emotional signal that something needs to change in one, or more, of three areas: your situation, your thinking, or your behavior.

Unfortunately, anger doesn't tell you what needs to change. In fact, it interferes with rational thinking. You can easily get swept away and direct your energy at a false target.

For this reason, dealing with anger is a two-step process:

1. Examine your anger to find out what needs to change and how to change it.

2. Change what is contributing to your anger.

Anger Is a Secondary Emotion

Anger has been called a "*secondary emotion*" because it is often triggered by underlying hurt or fear. Underneath your anger there may be the real emotion that you need to deal with and resolve.

Think about the common experience of feeling angry on the highway when another driver suddenly cuts you off, nearly causing an accident. In the split second before your anger, what are you feeling? Fear.

Think about what makes you angry with yourself, or with your children, or with other people. You may feel let down by them when they don't help with tasks you're not supposed to do because of lymphedema. You may worry about the consequences of others' actions. You may be hurt by comments by strangers or by healthcare professionals. You may feel like you are failing or being criticized when lymphedema isn't stable or because it can't be cured.

If you can change the situation, great, change it. But when you can't change the situation, you have to change your thinking and your actions because *staying chronically angry will harm you.* Staying angry—no matter how justified your anger—is not a good option. Use the Coping Suggestions on page 50.

Anger in My Life Worksheet

How big a role does anger play in your life with lymphedema? What triggers your anger? How you deal with anger? What emotions may be behind your anger?

Use Worksheet 4-1: **Anger in My Life** on page 51 to summarize what you have learned:

- Identify situations related to lymphedema that make you angry in the first column.

- Briefly summarize how you express your anger in the second column.

- Note the feelings that may be the cause of your anger in the third column.

Coping Suggestions:

Ask yourself:

☐ With whom am I angry?

☐ When do I get angry?

☐ What patterns do I see?

☐ Do I show any of the three patterns of problematic anger?

Explore what is underneath. If you think it may be fear, ask yourself what fears may be fueling your anger:

☐ Is anger my way of hiding fears triggered by lymphedema?

☐ Do I have fears about my health or my future because of lymphedema, or for some other reason?

☐ Do I worry about what will happen to my relationships if I acknowledge anger, or if I don't stay angry or if I don't stay on my guard all the time?

☐ When I get angry, am I protecting myself against something I fear such as failure, rejection, disappointment, etc.?

Review the key points about anger in this chapter. Apply these ideas.

Use the tools provided later in this book, especially thinking skills for dealing with any distressing emotion (Chapters 16) and communication skills (Chapter 18).

If fear fuels your anger, pay close attention to the next several chapters.

For example:

When Do I Get Angry?	What Do I Do?	What Other Feelings May Underlie My Anger?
My children and husband don't lift heavy items without being asked.	I lift more weight than I should and say nothing or else I yell & tell them they're selfish.	Sadness. Helplessness. Self-criticism. Fear that they think I'm a burden, selfish, or demanding.

Worksheet 4-1: Anger in My Life

When Do I Get Angry?	What Do I Do?	What Other Feelings May Underlie My Anger?

Now, turn to Worksheet 14-2: **My Emotional Challenges** on page 201 and complete the line for "Anger and resentment".

Resources

The Anger Control Workbook by Matthew McKay, PhD and Peter Rogers, PhD. New Harbinger Publications, 2000.

When Anger Hurts: Quieting the Storm Within by Matthew McKay, PhD, Peter Rogers, PhD, and Judith McKay, RN. New Harbinger Publications, 2003.

Anger Kills: 17 Strategies for Controlling the Hostility That Can Harm Your Heart by Redford Williams, MD and Virginia Williams, PhD. HarperPaperbacks, 1998.

Notes

1   **Winning the Race** by Nancy Brinker and Chriss Winston. Tapestry Press, 2001. p. 63

2   Research on interactions among anger, relationships, and health can be found in **Love & Survival: The Scientific Basis for the Healing Power of Intimacy** by Dean Ornish, MD. HarperCollins, 1998; **Healthy Pleasures** by Robert Ornstein, PhD and David Sobel, MD. Addison-Wesley, 1989; **Aging Well: Surprising Guideposts to a Happier Life from the Landmark Harvard Study of Adult Development** by George Vaillant, MD. Little, Brown and Company, 2002; and **Anger Kills: 17 Strategies for Controlling the Hostility That Can Harm Your Heart** by Redford Williams, MD and Virginia Williams, PhD. HarperPaperbacks, 1998.

3   **Anger Kills: 17 Strategies for Controlling the Hostility That Can Harm Your Heart** by Redford Williams, MD and Virginia Williams, PhD. HarperPaperbacks, 1998.

Chapter 5

Fear

Note:

- *Many of the ideas presented in this chapter also apply to the chapters on self-protective actions, worry, increased body focus, and self-consciousness.*

- *There are common themes in these chapters since many of these challenges include dealing with anxiety or fears. Even if you face only one of these challenges, consider reading the other chapters for a better understanding of the general ideas and principles.*

Normal Fear

Just as it is normal to feel angry about having lymphedema, it is normal to feel fear or to be scared. Feeling scared is not a sign of weakness; it is a sign of paying attention!

Congratulate yourself on being aware of your fear and on reading this book and this chapter. It contains some very reassuring information.

Stay with me and keep reading, even if you get a little scared. You can learn some incredibly helpful information.

The Importance of Courage

Let's face the bad news head-on. Lymphedema is not good news. It is legitimately scary. Its course is unpredictable. There are no guarantees or certainties. There is no cure and the possible complications are ugly.

Coping Suggestions:

Follow these four steps:

1. Admit that you're fearful and figure out what you are afraid may happen.

2. Get the relevant facts about what is actually happening, or is likely to happen. Don't let fear determine what you will do. You decide.

3. Act on the facts, even if this means doing something that scares you – in fact, especially if it means doing something that scares you.

4. Remind yourself that anxiety itself is unpleasant but harmless. Fear that is contradicted by facts is nothing but a false alarm.

What can you do when facing a scary situation like this?

Here is an example of applying these coping suggestions:

1. You think your swelling has increased. You notice that you feel tense and short of breath whenever you think about making a treatment appointment so you've been avoiding calling. You realize that you are scared your therapist will tell you that the swelling is much worse and will blame or shame you.

2. You start to measure your limb and record your measurements to actually discover whether and how much swelling is there. You remind yourself that in the past your therapist has been knowledgeable, supportive, accepting, and optimistic. You review the facts that maintaining treatment is important and helpful.

3. The measurements show some swelling. Even though this scares you even more and you don't want to think about it, you schedule an appointment.

4. You remind yourself that tense muscles, upset stomach, tight throat, shaky feelings, and feelings that you can't get a deep breath are all signs of anxiety and fear that you have experienced in the past. They are uncomfortable but not harmful.

Courage is not the absence of fear. Courage is going ahead and doing what you have to do while you are scared, despite being scared.

You don't control whether you feel frightened. You do control what you do in response to this feeling.

The Importance of Understanding Fear

Because feeling afraid is such an unpleasant experience, it is easy to take the wrong path when you are frightened. The information in this chapter will help keep you on track. You will learn:

- What happens when you feel anxious or afraid and why

- Ways that fear can cause problems in coping with lymphedema

- About resources and where to go for more information

The Fight-or-Flight Response

When we are afraid for any reason, our body responds physically with sympathetic nervous system arousal. This is known as the fight-or-flight response.

When this natural physical response goes off for reasons we don't understand, it is called an anxiety attack or a panic attack. Whether this response is mild or intense, whether you know what is causing it or not, the fight-or-flight response is natural, protective, and harmless.

Symptoms

The symptoms of fear vary from person to person and from time to time. A panic attack or anxiety attack is generally defined as four or more of these symptoms. They may seem to come out of the blue:

- Faster heartbeat

- Chest pressure, chest pain, or tightness in your chest

- Feeling short of breath or as if you're not getting enough air

- A choking feeling or lump in the throat

- Trembling or shaking

- Sweating
- Feeling unnaturally hot or cold
- Nausea, upset stomach, or gastrointestinal distress
- Dizziness or light-headedness
- Tingling or numbness
- Feeling as if you are cut off from yourself or as if what's around you isn't real

The fear response is definitely physical. It is definitely unpleasant. By itself, it is *not* harmful.[1]

Purpose

The fight-or-flight response was originally designed as a response to real physical danger. Each aspect of it has a life-saving purpose.

The fear response helped our ancestors survive in their dangerous world surrounded by predators. We inherited this response.

When the fight-or-flight response is triggered because we are physically threatened by real external danger, we don't worry about the symptoms because we know what caused them. In this situation, the symptoms don't feel dangerous to us.

Unfortunately, this response can be triggered when we are not facing a life-or-death confrontation. It sends a "false alarm." Even though we are not in danger, we feel afraid and so we have some or all of the physical sensations described above.

Triggers

What can trigger such false alarms? Many things can cause a fight-or-flight response. It can be set off by stress, by hormone fluctuations, or by some medications. It can be triggered by the emotion of fear itself or by fearful thoughts (conscious or unconscious). It can be activated by worry, by negative self-talk, or by unrealistic self-demands. It can be triggered because of things that happened in the past.

Why does this happen? This happens because the fight-or-flight response is activated by a very primitive part of the brain that is always on the lookout for danger. This part of our brain reacts automatically whenever it thinks there may be any type of threat. It doesn't stop to think. It doesn't evaluate the situation rationally. It reacts based on the information it receives – even if that information is wrong.

Summary

Lymphedema presents a threat. Your mind and body respond to threat by creating fear.

Fear is unpleasant. Fear reactions can be sudden or intense. They can even occur unexpectedly when you're asleep or relaxing. Fear reactions can be false alarms.

Fear *is* useful when, because of it, you seek out and act on accurate information about real threats facing you. Fear is *not* useful when you react to it by fearing things that are, in fact, not dangerous and by avoiding everything that scares you, regardless of the facts of the situation.

When you already have one disease, it is very common to fear that you have another disease when instead you are experiencing the fear reaction. Your first step, if you think a medical condition is causing your symptoms, is to talk to your physician or nurse. Get the facts.

If you learn that the problem is actually fear itself, use the coping suggestions in this chapter.

Problematic Fear: Panic, Phobias, and Avoidance

Problems occur when we mistakenly conclude that we are in danger even when we are not. We can either become frightened of the anxiety response itself or we can become frightened of the situation.

Fearing the symptoms of the fight-or-flight response is called *panic disorder*. Fearing a situation, even though it is not dangerous (or not as dangerous as we think) is called a phobia This chapter focuses on the experience of fear because that can occur in response to many worries. More specific worries and anxiety-provoking situations, such as dealing with the uncertainty of lymphedema, fear of infection, or worries about the future are covered in the chapters that follow.

Panic Disorder

The fight-or-flight reaction is very physical and pretty unpleasant. If you don't recognize that this reaction is protective and basically harmless, it is very easy to be frightened by it.

If you have had an unexpected panic or anxiety attack and now you are frightened and worry about having another one, you may have panic disorder. People with panic disorder fear anxiety. They may worry that the fear response symptoms mean something terrible. They may fear that they are having a heart attack or a stroke, fainting, dying, losing control, or going crazy. They may worry that something is medically wrong or that they are unable to function safely.

Coping Suggestions:

If you have had these symptoms and worry that you have some medical disease, talk to your healthcare professional. You may just be dealing with fear.

Phobias and Avoidance

A phobia is fear that:

- Is out of proportion to the actual danger **and**

- Causes marked distress or significant interference with normal functioning in some area of your life, such as work, relationships, or lymphedema care.

When you have a phobia, you believe that something is far more dangerous than it really is. You are extremely afraid when other people are not. The natural response to fear is to avoid what scares you, whether that is a place, an action, a situation, an object, a physical sensation, or a thought.

Unfortunately, this natural avoidance reaction maintains and strengthens fear. Avoidance makes it impossible for you to learn that what you fear is not as dangerous as you think it is. Avoidance makes it impossible for you to learn that you can safely cope with what you fear.

In other words, fear leads you to avoid. Avoidance causes you to continue to be afraid. The stronger your fear, the more you will want to avoid. And so on. A vicious cycle is established.

When you have lymphedema, fear can cause two types of problems unless you handle it correctly. First, fear can get in the way of effective lymphedema treatment. Second, fear makes it more difficult to master the emotional aspects of dealing with lymphedema. Here are some examples.

Fear of Fear

Fear of anxiety easily leads you to avoid anything that might trigger anxiety. Since reading about lymphedema can be anxiety-provoking for anyone, a strong fear of anxiety can make you reluctant to learn about lymphedema or to measure for signs of progress or problems.

Fear of anxiety can cause you to avoid situations or activities because you fear that having anxiety symptoms would be dangerous. Limiting your activities because of this fear is called agoraphobia.

Practically, if you fear leaving the house, driving a car, going to work, or going outside what feels like a safe comfort zone, you can find it difficult to keep medical appointments, consult with specialists, or attend lymphedema treatments.

Psychologically, confronting and overcoming the emotional aspects of lymphedema takes courage. You need to be willing to face fear.

Social Fears

Many people have some discomfort at the prospect of being criticized or meeting strangers. If this fear is particularly strong, however, it may be what is called social phobia. The newer name is social anxiety disorder.

Because lymphedema is often visible and draws the attention of others, you may be more at risk of being anxious in social situations. Such anxiety can be troublesome by making it more difficult to deal with normal self-consciousness (see Chapter 9: Self-Consciousness) or with others' common reactions (see Chapter 10: Others' Reactions).

If you strongly fear embarrassment, you may avoid situations where you could be the focus of attention or where you would interact with other people. As a result, you may not attend lymphedema educational classes or support groups.

A fear of other people observing or judging you can make you miss appointments, show up late, or not report problems. It can make you unwilling to ask questions or to say no. It can make it harder to get your needs met by your healthcare professionals and others in your life.

Successful living with lymphedema involves being willing to speak up at times. You succeed when you find ways to reach out to others who can help.

Specific Fears

Sometimes you aren't afraid of fear itself or of other people's reactions. Sometimes you are afraid because the situation itself seems dangerous. When you think a specific thing, or object, or situation, is more dangerous than it is and when your fear is very distressing or when it disrupts your life, then this can be called a specific phobia.

Specific phobias are sometimes named for the focus of the fear. For example, claustrophobia is the name for a specific phobia of enclosed spaces. Fear of enclosed spaces, fear of heights, fear of planes, fear of dentists, and fear of medical procedures are all rather common specific phobias.

Such fears can compromise your treatment. You may avoid medical appointments because the examination or treatment room seems too enclosed or because the office is in a building or on a floor that seems too high. You may avoid important lab tests because of a phobia of needles or blood.

Claustrophobia can be a particularly troublesome fear when you have lymphedema. If you have claustrophobia, being bandaged or wearing your compression garment can make you feel like you can't breathe. You can feel trapped or terrified.

This experience is different from being a little anxious about whether you are bandaging properly or whether the compression garment will be effective. This normal fear doesn't interfere with treatment; claustrophobia, if untreated, can lead you to stop bandaging or wearing your compression garment. You then stay afraid of compression and your lymphedema worsens because it is not being effectively controlled.

Summary

You *should* fear things that are really dangerous. When appropriately triggered by a real threat, fear and anxiety serve a helpful purpose. They alert you so that you can avoid danger and harm.

Fear of the consequences of untreated lymphedema is helpful if this fear leads you to take reasonable actions to protect your health and improve your quality of life. It is not helpful if your fear leads you to avoid taking protective action. What can you do if fear is a problem?

Face Your Fears

Face your fears. Avoiding what you fear is problematic for two reasons:

- **First,** it keeps you from learning that what you fear is not as dangerous or overwhelming as you think.

- **Second,** escaping or avoiding what your fear takes away opportunities to cope despite fear, to learn new skills, and to develop more self-confidence.

Fear is common. Nobody likes getting shots or having blood drawn. Doctor or dentist appointments are not considered fun. Many of us dislike these things, worry about them, or get a little anxious beforehand. But avoiding needed tests can keep you from getting good care.

What To Do

You can reduce and handle your anxiety response. Use these coping suggestions.

Coping Suggestions:

Expect the fear and label it as the false alarm it is.

Use slow, deep, steady breathing to tolerate the fear.

Remember to follow the four coping suggestions on page 54.

If you fear the physical anxiety response itself, consider reading **Mastery of Your Anxiety and Panic** (see **Resources** below).

If you have social anxiety, consider reading **Dying of Embarrassment: Help for Social Anxiety and Phobia** and/or **The Shyness and Social Anxiety Workbook** (see **Resources** on page 64).

If you have specific fears such as claustrophobia, consider reading **Mastery of Your Specific Phobia** (see **Resources** below).

Use the skills in Section IV: **Tools for Change.**

Consider talking to a mental health professional with training and skill in treating phobias and panic. Specific cognitive-behavioral treatments are extremely effective.

If fear is only an occasional problem when you need dental care or a lab test, ask your physician about a fast-acting anti-anxiety medication.

Fear and Its Impact Worksheet

You have learned about the fight-or-flight response and about ways fear can disrupt your life with lymphedema. Remember that fear is meant to be helpful.

Helpful fear is fear that is proportional to the actual danger and which motivates you to take appropriate action to prevent harm. A good example would be having a healthy fear of getting a cut on your arm that is affected by lymphedema and taking reasonable precautions. The issue of deciding what precautions are reasonable is discussed in Chapter 6: Being Self-Protective.

You want your level of fear to be in line with reality. You may need to learn to be less afraid of some things that aren't really dangerous. Or you may need to learn to be more respectful of some things, such as the complications of lymphedema, so that fear encourages you to take reasonable protective actions to prevent complications and improve your health and functioning.

Use Worksheet 5-1: **Fear and Its Impact** on page 65 to write down what you have learned about the role of anxiety and fear in your life:

1. Think about your answers to the questions in this chapter, specifically what makes you afraid and what you fear might happen. Write your answers in the left column.

2. Think about how these fears affect your life and, specifically, their positive or negative impact on your lymphedema. Write these answers in the right hand column.

Now, turn to Worksheet 14-2: **My Emotional Challenges** on page 201 and complete the line for "Fear."

Resources

Dying of Embarrassment: Help for Social Anxiety and Phobia by Barbara Markway, PhD, Cheryl Carmin, PhD, C. Alec Pollard, PhD, and Teresa Flynn, PhD. New Harbinger Publications, 1992.

The Shyness and Social Anxiety Workbook: Proven Techniques for Overcoming Your Fears by Martin Antony, PhD and Richard Swinson, MD. New Harbinger Publications, 2000.

Mastery of Your Anxiety and Panic - Third Edition (MAP III), Client Workbook by David Barlow, PhD and Michelle Craske, PhD. Oxford University Press, 2000.

The Agoraphobia Workbook: A Comprehensive Program to End Your Fear of Symptom Attacks by C. Alec Pollard, PhD and Elke Zuercher-White, PhD. New Harbinger Publications, 2003.

An End to Panic: Breakthrough Techniques for Overcoming Panic Disorder, 2nd Ed by Elke Zuercher-White, PhD. New Harbinger Publications, 2000.

Mastery of Your Specific Phobia, Client Workbook by Martin Antony, PhD, Michelle Craske, PhD, and David Barlow, PhD. Oxford University Press, 1995.

Worksheet 5-1: Fear and Its Impacts

When Do I Become Anxious? What Do I Fear May Happen?	What Impact Does Fear Have on My Life, Happiness, or Lymphedema Care?

Notes

1   Since similar symptoms *can* be caused by medical problems such as
thyroid disease, it is always a good idea to discuss your symptoms with
your primary healthcare professional. This is especially true if you fear
these bodily sensations.

Chapter 6

Being Self-Protective

Life with lymphedema is filled with many cautions, precautions, and self-management responsibilities. You fear that you might do something to harm the swollen area of your body. You wonder, *"What's safe? What's not?"* The emotional challenge here is finding the right amount of self-protection for you.

Normal Increased Self-Protection

The rules of daily life change when you get lymphedema. Activities that previously were safe may suddenly be hazardous. Things you did without thinking, such as gardening barehanded in the hot sun or walking barefoot, may now require that you take precautions—or avoid them entirely.

Actions you previously thought could be ignored or postponed, such as healthy eating and exercising regularly, are now more urgently important. Increased self-protection is a normal, healthy, adaptive response to lymphedema.

Of course, normal, healthy, and adaptive does not mean easy. Being forced to change what you do is aggravating. Uncertainty makes these changes harder.

Uncertainty

You can feel confused, frustrated, and unsettled when you hear different opinions about what is, or is not, an appropriate level of self-protection. How do you decide what is appropriate? Why is there uncertainty? Why aren't there clear, unchanging rules for everyone?

You will encounter uncertainty for several reasons:

1. Specific protective actions vary somewhat from person to person. You may bandage daily, while your friend uses compression garments.

2. What you can do may vary from day to day based on changes in the current state of your lymphedema, the weather, your weight, your overall physical condition, and other factors. Clothing and jewelry that you wore yesterday may be too tight today. The exercise that was strenuous last month may not give you enough of a workout now that you are stronger.

3. Experts in the field offer differing opinions about specifics of treatment and about what are appropriate precautions and safe activities. Plus, as more is learned and better treatments develop, recommendations about what to do, or not to do, will change.

Every day you must decide what you can do safely and what may be risky. Some situations are clear. For example, don't work in a razor blade factory or use your bare hands to handle roses with thorns.

Many other situations are unclear. *"How much risk do I face if I fly? Can I garden? Do I take hikes in the woods as long as I use insect repellent? Can I resume my favorite sport? How hard can I exercise and what exercise can I do?"*

Informed, Effective Self-Protection

People don't like feeling uncertain, especially about things that are important to us. Our natural human response is look for ways to reduce uncertainty. We like to feel in control. We want predictability.

The effective response to uncertainty is to seek out knowledge, look for patterns, learn over time what does and doesn't work for you, and change what you do based on the information you've gained. You are doing that by reading this book.

Getting a chronic illness like lymphedema is rather like suddenly finding yourself in a new country. Your job is to create your own living-well-with-lymphedema map.

While mapping out this new territory, you try to determine what is safe and what's not, what is important to do or to avoid and what's irrelevant and can be ignored. You want to create a map that is as accurate and useful as

Coping Suggestions:

Talk to healthcare professionals, lymphedema organizations, and support groups to learn from their knowledge and experience.

Read books, such as **Living Well With Lymphedema,** which offer practical advice based on the most current knowledge.

See **Resources** at the end of this chapter for websites that provide reliable, up-to-date information.

Learn the signs of a lymphedema emergency so you can judge if a scratch is becoming infected.

Plan ahead and be prepared. For example, if you will be traveling, decide what self-protection steps to take (such as using compression if you are flying) and ask your doctor if you should carry medication in case of infection.

Accept that there is no one best way to protect oneself. Each person is different.

Learn how to monitor your lymphedema and do so. For example, if lymphedema affects your arm, have your therapist show you how to measure your arm. By measuring at home, you track your progress and measure the effectiveness of your actions.

Base your self-protection decisions on facts. Look for patterns. See which activities help, or worsen, your lymphedema. If you are uncertain about a certain activity, you might particularly notice changes in size, shape, texture, heaviness, or tenderness before and afterward.

Balance risks, benefits, and quality of life.

possible. And you need to follow your map and actively update it from your experiences.

Problematic Responses to the Need for Self-Protection

What can go wrong in confronting the challenge of being more protective of your body in the face of uncertainty? Two problematic responses to this issue will be discussed here:

- Refusing to deal with the problem by denying its existence or

- Becoming irrationally over-restrictive.

Juan's Story

My leg got badly injured when I crashed my mountain bike last year. It was a nasty infected wound that required hospitalization and physical therapy and left major scarring. I thought it had healed but the leg kept getting swollen and uncomfortable. When I went to the doctor, she explained it was lymphedema.

Lympha-what? That sounded so awful that it's like I stopped listening. My gut reaction was that my leg was going to swell up so that I couldn't walk, and it would eventually have to be amputated.

In hindsight, I was paralyzed by fear. She made an appointment with a lymphedema therapist but I didn't keep it. I didn't want to hear more bad news. I was afraid I would overstress the leg by using it. I quit shooting hoops with the guys. Instead I became a couch potato or played computer games. My buddies just wouldn't give up though. They kept asking what had to be done. They even researched lymphedema on the Internet and kept bugging me to get help.

I finally got up my courage to see the lymphedema therapist and he managed to break that headlock that fear had on me. Together we got started on my lymphedema treatment. Today my only question is, *"Why did I ever let fear take over? It was ruining my life."*

Denying or Rebelling

One response to the discomfort of uncertainty and the need for change is to simply refuse to deal with it. You deny any need for increased self-protection. You act as if lymphedema doesn't exist.

Here are warning signals that you are denying or rebelling against the need for increased self-protection:

☐ I avoid self-protective measures—despite medical advice. I pretend they're not necessary or don't apply to me.

☐ I see no need to make changes. Lymphedema is not serious.

☐ I ignore swelling and warning sensations.

☐ I admit that a problem exists, but don't change my behavior—no matter what.

☐ I deliberately take risks. Not only do I refuse to protect myself, I actively put myself in danger.

If you checked off **any** of the boxes above, you are acting this way for a reason. Consider what thoughts and emotions are behind your actions. These actions are keeping you from better health and improved quality of life.

Coping Suggestions:

If you aren't sure you want to change, read about precontemplation, the first step in the five steps of change in Chapter 15, starting on page 207.

If you see a need to change your actions, identify what you are thinking or feeling and then read or reread the relevant chapters. For example:

- If you are acting this way out of anger, see Chapter 4.
- If you feel hopeless or overwhelmed, reread Chapter 2 and Chapter 3.

If reality problems, like lack of money, are causing you to act this way, follow the suggestions given in Chapter 13: Current Stress.

Becoming Overly Restrictive

The other problematic response to this challenge is becoming overly or irrationally restrictive. Your self-protective actions may be too limiting and extreme. They may not make sense.

The symptoms of lymphedema can wax and wane, despite your best efforts. This is confusing and sometimes you think you see connections where they don't really exist. If this happens, you can develop what are called superstitious behaviors.

This means you start to do things to protect yourself that are based on false assumptions and superstition, not based on facts and logic. Superstitious behaviors are actions that don't really change anything.

Sometimes superstitious behavior is not a big deal. You may want to park in the "lucky" parking space at the treatment center. A kiss from your partner may help you feel safer before going to the doctor. Common examples from everyday life include the baseball pitcher who touches his cap in a certain "lucky" way before every pitch and the performers who urge each other to "break a leg" before going on stage.

Superstitious behaviors cause difficulties when they take up lots of time or energy or interfere with our functioning. If this sounds like you, you may want to learn about an anxiety problem called obsessive-compulsive disorder (OCD).

Obsessive-Compulsive Behavior

In this context, the word **obsessive** means that distressing or frightening thoughts come into your mind repeatedly even if you don't want them. These thoughts can be hard to stop or ignore. They are not appropriate worry about real-life problems or a reliving of past traumatic events.

The word **compulsive** means that you feel you have to do something to avoid harm. This can be an action you need to take or avoid or it can be a thought you need to think or avoid thinking. When your thoughts and actions are particularly troublesome, they may be called obsessive-compulsive disorder.

Obsessive-compulsive disorder is an anxiety problem. Like all anxiety problems, it can be triggered or worsened by stress, by uncertainty, or by past trauma—and most people with lymphedema are dealing with all three!

How Can I Tell the Difference?

Lymphedema means that you *do* need to pay more attention to your health and your daily activities than you did and that you *do* need to do things differently. How might obsessive-compulsive disorder look different from conscientious coping with lymphedema?

Ask yourself these questions:

- Am I spending an excessive amount of time on self-management? For example, do I spend much more time on self-massage than my therapist recommends? Do I have to bandage and rebandage a specific number of times—not how my therapist showed me.

- Am I doing or avoiding activities that lymphedema experts say do not have to be done or avoided? For example, do I restrict protein or fluids in my diet in an attempt to cure my lymphedema? Am I avoiding all lifting and exercise? Am I avoiding going outside at any time for fear of getting a mosquito bite?

- Am I saving things? Do I keep old bandages that are no longer effective? Do I hoard left-over antibiotics long after their expiration date?

- When I explain the reason for my behavior, does it make no sense to people who are knowledgeable about lymphedema? What do my lymphedema therapist and knowledgeable members of my healthcare team tell me when I talk about my actions? Am I hiding what I do because I am ashamed or because I expect they'll think it's "weird" or "crazy"?

- Am I so terrified of any risk at all that I am spending much more time on precautions than is recommended? Do I spend hours each day inspecting the affected tissues for signs of an infection or a break in the skin? Do I repeatedly ask other people to check over and over again even when everything looks fine?

- Are my protective behaviors not connected logically to the harm they are supposed to prevent? Are certain bandages 'safe'? Do the boxes all have to be facing the same way? Do I have to have a 'lucky' number of bandages and avoid an 'unlucky' number? Do I fear that thinking about a complication will cause it and so I desperately try not to have such thoughts?

- Are my protective behaviors actually putting me more at risk? For example, washing with reasonable frequency using mild soap is recommended. Do I instead wash the affected tissues with harsh cleansers that leave the skin rough, reddened, or chafed? Do I wash so often or for so long that the skin becomes chapped? These actions open a pathway for infection. Do I avoid so many activities trying to protect myself that I don't get sufficient exercise?

If you answered yes to any of the above questions, the changes you are making may be causing you more harm than good. Consider reading one of the self-help books for obsessive-compulsive disorder listed in the **Resources** section at the end of this chapter. You may find some of the self-help skills very useful.

Depending on how distressing or disruptive this problematic self-protective response is, you may want to consult a mental health professional; ideally someone who is a specialist in anxiety disorders and has experience treating OCD. No matter how severe, how extensive, or how long-standing your symptoms, research clearly shows that you can get significant relief from treatment.

What Should I Do?

You don't want to take too few precautions; you don't want to take too many precautions; you don't want to engage in superstitious behavior and take useless, unhelpful actions. How do you decide?

Which sources of advice should you trust? How do you evaluate if the basis for the suggestion or the source of the suggested action is credible? The coping suggestions on page 75 can help.

The Bottom Line

When you get advice from credible sources you trust, consider doing what is advised. Discover which self-protective actions give you the best results.

Build on what works. Change or discard what doesn't work. By following these two guidelines, you should have increased self-protection that is effective and appropriate: not too little; not too much.

Coping Suggestions:

☐ A trained and experienced lymphedema therapist who treats you and whose past suggestions have been helpful would be considered a credible source of advice.

☐ Suggestions based on knowledge and logic or suggestions that stem from your personal experience would also be credible.

☐ Ask questions such as, *"Is a suggestion supported by actual evidence, not just stories?" "Is the suggestion logical and consistent with what I know about lymphedema?" "Is the source of the suggestions respected by qualified lymphedema experts?" "What experience, training, knowledge, or success rate does the source of the information have?" "How can I verify this?"*

☐ When getting information from the Internet, look for websites displaying the HONcode logo. This logo verifies that the website complies with the Health On the Net principles (www.hon.ch) designed to increase the accuracy, objectivity, and trustworthiness of health information offered on the Internet.

Increased Self-Protection in My Life Worksheet

Think about what you have learned so far. Use Worksheet 6-1: Increased Self-Protection in My Life to review the impact of self-protective actions on your life. You may need to do more. Or you may be able to do less.

1. In the first column, summarize your current self-protection actions. List specific things you do to prevent or treat lymphedema flare-ups.

2. In the second column, write down the source of each suggestion and how credible and knowledgeable you think the source is. See the coping suggestions above on ways to evaluate sources of suggestions.

3. In the third column, evaluate your results. How do you, or will you, measure the results? How well are your protective actions working? Are you happy with them? If you are unhappy with the results, think about what you will change and write down your ideas in the first column. Redo the worksheet deciding how you'll decide if the idea is credible and how you will measure its effectiveness.

Think about your answers to the questions and worksheet in this chapter. Review your answers and what you have learned.

Now, turn to Worksheet 14-2: **My Emotional Challenges** on page 201 and complete the line for "Increased Self-Protection."

Worksheet 6-1: Increased Self-Protection in My Life

Self-Protection Actions	Source – How Credible?	Results

Resources

Effective Self-Protection Resources

Living Well With Lymphedema by Ann Ehrlich, Alma Vinjé-Harrewijn, PT, CLT and Elizabeth McMahon, PhD. Lymph Notes, 2005.

Lymphedema: A Breast Cancer Patient's Guide To Prevention And Healing by Jeannie Burt and Gwen White. Publishers Group West, 1999.

Coping With Lymphedema by Joan Swirsky and Dianne Nannery. Avery Publishing Group, 1998.

www.LymphNotes.com - an online resource and support group for persons with lymphedema and their family members and for lymphedema therapists. It also provides information about lymphedema, treatment resources, and support groups.

www.lymphnet.org - website of the National Lymphedema Network, a nonprofit organization providing information about lymphedema, treatment resources, and support groups.

Obsessive-Compulsive Disorder Resources

Stop Obsessing: How to Overcome Your Obsessions and Compulsions by Edna Foa, PhD and Reid Wilson, PhD. Bantam Books, 2001.

Brain Lock: Free Yourself from Obsessive-Compulsive Behavior by Jeffrey Schwartz, MD. Regan Books, 1997.

Obsessive-Compulsive Disorders: A Complete Guide to Getting Well and Staying Well by Fred Penzel. Oxford University Press, 2000.

Chapter 7

Worry and Uncertainty

Lymphedema brings risks and uncertainty. Worry is a natural consequence.

The capacity to worry about realistic dangers is essential to human survival. Because you can imagine likely problems before they occur, you can take steps to avoid, minimize, or cope with them.

This is a triumph of human capacity and creativity and something of which you should be very proud. You will use this strength to cope successfully with lymphedema.

Normal Worry

It is normal and natural to worry when you are diagnosed with lymphedema. You worry about what it means. You wonder about the future. Your lymphedema symptoms vary which creates uncertainty. A natural response to uncertainty is to worry, to ask *"What if...?"*

When worry about lymphedema leads you to take good care of yourself, it is helpful and healthy.

Signs of Helpful Worry

Signs that your worry is normal, healthy, and adaptive include:

☐ You worry about dangers that are likely.

☐ Your worries are based on facts and are not exaggerated.

☐ Your worry leads you to take action that decrease the danger.

☐   Your level of worry lessens after you take action.

How many of the above describe you? If you checked every box, congratulate yourself and keep up the good work.

Look back at the list of signs of helpful worry. Were there any of those that do not describe you? Which ones? Keep your answers in mind as you read the rest of this chapter.

Coping Suggestions:

Continue to take actions to treat your lymphedema and protect yourself that are effective and are recommended by credible sources. Read Chapter 6: Increased Self-Protection if you have questions about what appropriate self-protection is or how to decide if a source of advice is credible.

If you are *not* taking appropriate actions, notice the thoughts and emotions that are stopping you. Then read the relevant emotional challenge chapter that addresses those thoughts and emotions. For example, if you are angry read Chapter 4, if you are scared read Chapter 5, etc. Chapter 15: The Five Steps of Change may also help.

Your ability to worry is a reflection of your intelligence, your foresight, and your imagination. Worry is a powerful tool and, like every powerful tool, can help or harm.

Problematic Worry

Sometimes, worry seems to take on a life of its own. It is as if your brain gets stuck in worry mode. When this happens, worrying creates problems.

Over-Worrying about Lymphedema

“   Worry, Worry, Worry
I can't ever relax. I always worry about infection and lymph-edema. My therapist says I'm doing fine, but I can't get those pictures of huge swollen legs out of my mind. What if that's   **”**
me? What if treatment stops working?

You may wonder if you are over-worrying about lymphedema. Here are some signs that this may be happening:

☐ Does your brain keep imagining lymphedema problems over and over and never moves on to solutions?

☐ Do you see danger lurking where others with lymphedema don't?

☐ Do you have to forestall and plan in detail for every conceivable lymphedema-related danger, however unlikely.

☐ Does daily life seem is filled with threats of all kinds, above and beyond the recommended precautions?

☐ Do you continue to be distressed by worry about lymphedema even though you are taking realistic self-protective actions and follow self-management guidelines?

☐ Does your level of worry and concern remain high and not decrease despite evidence that treatment is working?

☐ Do you feel you worry too much about lymphedema, but you can't seem to stop?

How many of the above describe you? If you checked one or more of the boxes, you may indeed be over-worrying about lymphedema. This can be distressing, discouraging, and unhelpful.

General Over-Worrying

Sometimes people generally worry too much about everything or have a lot of trouble accepting uncertainty. Dealing with lymphedema is harder and more exhausting if you usually over-worry.

For some people, this has been a problem since childhood. People sometimes describe themselves as being "a worrier" or a "worry wart" or feel as if they have a "worry machine" inside that they can't turn off.

If you have checked with your medical doctor to make sure that your tension and worry are not caused by a medical condition or medication, you may have anxiety that has spread or "generalized" to many different areas.

How many of these describe you? Check each the signs that apply:

☐ Have you been worrying too much, more days than not, for 6 months or longer about many different things?

☐ Do you find it difficult to control the worry?

☐ Does worry make you edgy, irritable, or easily tired?

☐ Does worry interfere with sleep or concentration?

☐ Are your muscles tense?

☐ Is worrying upsetting you or interfering with your functioning?

If you checked two or more of the boxes, you may have what is called generalized anxiety disorder (sometimes known as GAD).

To treat generalized anxiety disorder, you learn to challenge your beliefs about the accuracy or usefulness of worry and to tolerate worry and uncertainty. Many of the medicines that are effective for depression or other anxiety problems help this problem as well.

Reducing Over-Worry

Start with the coping suggestions on page 83 and use skills from the rest of this book as you need them. The suggestions will help you fight back against worry. They can help with any troublesome worry, whether you worry about one area of your life or many.

Worry and Its Impact on Your Life

Review your answers to these three checklists and ask yourself:

☐ Do I have helpful worry? I checked _____ out of 4 signs of "Helpful Worry" on page 79.

☐ Do I over-worry about lymphedema? I checked _____ out of 4 signs of "Over-Worry about Lymphedema" on page 81.

☐ Do I over-worry in general? I checked ___ out of 6 signs of "Generalized Worry" on this page.

Coping Suggestions:

Turn to the facts to decide whether your worries are realistic. How probable or likely are they? Out of all the times you have worried, how often has what you worried about actually happened and how bad has it been?

Review the facts. Base your actions upon the facts.

Challenge the usefulness of worrying. Ask yourself if it actually helps. Is it distressing you rather than protecting you?

Restrict the time you spend worrying, arguing with the worries, or trying to stop worrying. See page 243 in Chapter 16 for details on how to schedule "worry time".

Accept worries when they arise - without acting on them. When worry conflicts with fact, act on what the facts tell you, not what the worry says.

Acknowledge and accept the fact that you must live with uncertainty. Chapter 6: Increased Self-Protection discusses this in more depth.

Deliberately practice tolerating uncertainty. Remind yourself that nothing can really guarantee safety or certainty and yet most people tolerate this and live happily.

Chapter 16: Thinking Skills provides additional tools to help you apply these coping suggestions.

To learn more about self-help techniques and psychotherapy approaches for reducing over-worry, see Resources at the end of this chapter.

Worry and the Facts Worksheet

Compare your worries against the facts. Are you worrying too much? Too little? Do the facts support your worries?

In Worksheet 7-1:

* Write each of your major worries in the first column.

* For each worry, summarize the facts in the second column.

* Compare each worry to the facts and write your answer in the third column.

Here is an example:

What My Worries Tell Me	What The Facts Tell Me	Do The Facts Suggest I Should Worry More Or Less?
Lymphedema is a bad problem. *What if it gets worse and worse?* *What if I get infection that can't be treated?*	*Lymphedema is serious but mine mostly worsens only if I don't follow my therapist's recommendations. I only had 1 infection since I started treatment & it responded to antibiotics. I know the signs of infection and follow the recommended precautions. My swelling has gone way down. Nothing is certain in life, but I'm doing pretty good. I'll just cope with whatever comes, when it comes. Extra worry doesn't help.*	*I don't have to worry this much.*

Worksheet 7-1: Worry and the Facts

What My Worries Tell Me	What The Facts Tell Me	Do The Facts Suggest I Should Worry More Or Less?

Actions, Effects, and Worry Level Worksheet

You might respond to worry by learning the signs of infection, knowing appropriate first aid to take when you get a cut, and carrying antibiotics.

What actions do you take to avoid harm? What is the effect of these actions on your life? Are your actions consistent with the facts and therefore likely to protect you?

What is the effect of these actions on your level of worry? Do you worry less or do you continue to worry no matter what you do?

In Worksheet 7-2:

- Write each action you take due to worry in the first column.

- Summarize the effect of these actions on your life in the second column.

- Evaluate the effect of your actions on your worry in the third column.

Here is an example:

Action Taken Due To Worry	Effect On My Life	Effect on My Worry
I carry antibiotics, wrap my limb when I fly, and measure to check for swelling.	*I travel again and go on trips.* *I am freer.*	*Less worried.* *More confident.*

Think about your answers to the questions and worksheets in this chapter. Review your answers and what you have learned.

Now, turn to Worksheet 14-2: **My Emotional Challenges** on page 201 and complete the line for "Worry".

Worksheet 7-2: Actions, Effects, and Worry Level

Action Taken Due To Worry	Effect On My Life	Effect on My Worry

Resources

Mastery of Your Anxiety and Worry, Client Manual by Richard Zinbarg, PhD, Michelle Craske, PhD, and David Barlow, PhD. Oxford University Press, 1992.

Overcoming Generalized Anxiety Disorder – Client Manual by John White, PhD. New Harbinger, 1999.

Stop Obsessing: How to Overcome Your Obsessions and Compulsions by Edna Foa, PhD and Reid Wilson, PhD. Bantam Books, 2001. (Chapter 5 deals with repetitive, intrusive worries.)

Chapter **8:**

Focusing On Your Body

Before developing lymphedema, you may not have thought about your body very much. Almost certainly you didn't think about your lymphatic system. You could take for granted that your body handled the flow and drainage of lymph on its own.

The luxury of that unawareness is now a thing of the past. Your body needs your conscious attention. Your body needs your help.

Normal Increased Body Focus

Knowing when and how to help your body requires that you focus more on minor bodily changes. For people without lymphedema, getting a cut, running a fever, or having some pain are just minor nuisances, something they barely notice. When you have lymphedema, you have a more challenging task.

You need heightened awareness of minor variations within your body. Tingling or heaviness may signal increased swelling before it is visible. Responding to such signals lets you increase your self-care and minimize the symptoms.

Noticing and immediately treating an insect bite may prevent, or quickly and successfully treat, worsened lymphedema and infection. Ignoring the bite can result in serious infection.

Becoming attentive to minor changes in limb size and sensation lets you protect your body. You can take actions that help your lymph system function most effectively. An increased focus on your body is a normal, necessary, and healthy response to lymphedema.

Finding the Balance Between Two Extremes

However, as with all the emotional challenges brought into your life by this condition, an increased focus on your body can also lead to unintended problems. And, as with so much of what you are learning, the key is to find a balance between two extremes.

On the one hand, ignoring your body and your lymphedema is courting disaster. It is like walking along the edge of a cliff with your eyes closed. You make yourself vulnerable to serious problems that could have been avoided entirely or minimized.

On the other hand, focusing on your body and your lymphedema to the exclusion of other things unnecessarily restricts your life. It is like spending your life cowering behind bars in a cage. You may avoid disaster, but you also avoid joy, activity, and growth. You wither away emotionally and physically.

What Can You Do?

It is true that life is different since you developed lymphedema. That's a fact. You don't have the carefree freedom you may have known before.

At the same time, every bodily sensation is **not** a sign of impending disaster or physical disability. These coping suggestions can help you develop a healthy and helpful increased body focus.

Coping Suggestions:

Inform yourself about the early warning signs of a lymphedema flare-up. See **Resources** for Self-Protection on page 78.

Learn the warning signs of infection.

Follow the self-care actions recommended by reliable sources.

Don't automatically assume that you are incapable of doing things. Be willing to push yourself a little beyond your comfort zone. Don't give in. Don't give up. Don't assume the worst.

Track your progress and do more of what works. You may surprise yourself with the results!

Women breast cancer survivors throughout the world who have, or who are at risk for, lymphedema are increasing their endurance and strength by careful training and are participating in dragon boat races.[1] People with lymphedema go sailing and scuba diving. They do yoga and water exercises. Research is planned to explore whether strength training would help lymphedema.[2]

Your body may be able to do more than you think, especially if you build up to it gradually. Talk to your lymphedema therapist.

Mind-Body Interactions

As discussed, focusing on your body is important and necessary. And yet, focusing on your body can create problems because the mind and the body interact in complicated, automatic, and unconscious ways.

You may have noticed that the strength of physical sensations in your body increases when you pay attention to them. For example, you are probably most aware of the tightness of the bandages when you are wrapping and carefully adjusting the tension. You are probably less aware of those sensations when you are watching an exciting movie or in the midst of an interesting conversation or activity.

Your body is constantly creating thousands of sensations. This is true for all of us—you, me, everyone. You would be overwhelmed if you had to be consciously aware of each sensation, each tiny change in posture, in temperature, in heartbeat, in touch, in background noise, and so on and so on.

To protect yourself from being overwhelmed, there is a part of your mind located in the lower part of the brain that automatically notices, filters, and sorts through the constant incoming noise of physical sensations. Its job is to sort out the important information signals from the background noise.

Think of this part of the brain as being like the executive assistant for a high-powered boss of an enormously complicated business. The boss can't deal with every piece of junk mail and every phone call. The assistant sorts and discards what seems unimportant and calls the boss' attention to what is important.

The boss only knows about information that the assistant passes on. And the boss assumes that if the information gets passed on, it is probably important.

In just the same way, this lower level of your mind sorts through what it thinks is important and what it thinks isn't. Only the information it decides is important gets through to your conscious awareness.

Sometimes your lower brain comes to the right conclusion. When this is the case, we automatically notice sensations that are important. We automatically ignore sensations that are physically present but that are meaningless or harmless.

Sometimes your lower brain comes to the wrong conclusion about whether something is important enough to get your conscious attention. It can make one of two errors:

- **Ignoring sensations that signal illness.** By educating yourself about lymphedema and following the coping suggestions above, you minimize the chance of this error.

- **Becoming overly vigilant and reacting to meaningless or harmless sensations.** This happens automatically, below conscious awareness. Unfortunately, a vicious cycle can then begin. As you start to consciously notice and monitor these bodily sensations on the higher level of your mind, your attention causes these physical sensations to get stronger and/or to occur more often. This increase in strength or frequency of sensations occurs because you are paying attention, not because something is wrong.

Let's repeat this important fact. How strong a physical sensation feels partly depends on how much attention you are paying to it. Think of examples from your own life. Will you be more aware of a headache or the heaviness of lymphedema during an interesting TV drama or when you are lying in bed with nothing to distract you?

How strong a physical sensation is and how consciously aware you are of it are also both influenced by whether the executive assistant, sorting part of your mind thinks the sensation is dangerous or important. Obviously, the assistant is going to try harder, louder, and more often to get the boss to pay attention to crucial information.

Think of examples from your own life. If you have what you believe is a common, harmless, tension headache, you may not pay a great deal of attention to it. The level of pain and awareness may fluctuate. On the other hand, if you fear that the headache is a sign of a brain tumor, you are more aware of the pain and you experience more pain.

Problematic Body Focus

What this means for you is that you can misinterpret the importance and meaning of physical symptoms. Your body's sensations will vary depending on your beliefs about them. Here are two common patterns that can signal problematic body focus.

Problematic Body Focus 1: Symptoms Equal Disease

One type of problematic body focus is when you come to believe that every physical sensation or change is a sign of disease. You find yourself constantly worrying that your bodily symptoms mean you have a terrible disease, even when the facts are reassuring. This is a form of over-worry where the worry is confined to worry about your health. You find yourself overly focused on your body and its sensations.

Signs that this may be an issue for you are:

☐ Your worries focus on bodily symptoms and disease and your health fears distress, upset, and disturb you. You do not worry about other issues. If you worry too much about all kinds of things, reread Chapter 7.

☐ Your health fears are not supported by facts, and yet the fear does not go away.

☐ Reassuring test results, examinations, or information only relieve your fear temporarily.

☐ At least some of the time, you think you may be worrying without cause, but you find it hard to believe this.

If you checked *any* of the boxes above, this type of problematic body focus is probably an issue for you. Read the rest of this chapter carefully and use the ideas and suggestions.

If you checked *all* of the boxes above, you may be wrestling with excessive health fear, which is sometimes known as *hypochondriasis*. This type of negative focus on your body can cause emotional pain, disrupt your life, and derail your attention from coping with lymphedema and focusing on symptoms that are actually important.

You may be flooded with fears of disease. Your tests come back normal. Health professionals you trust aren't worried about your symptoms. It has been six months or more and the things you fear haven't happened. Yet you can't shake the idea that there's a disease that hasn't been found.

Perhaps you are temporarily reassured when findings are normal, but the fear returns. Emotionally, you can't shake the fear that you have an undiagnosed disease. You may keep worrying about one disease in particular or you may worry about different diseases, one after another.

Perhaps, no matter what you do, you can't hold on to a feeling of reassurance or safety. You keep calling your health care professionals. You worry that you didn't tell them something crucial or that they didn't listen, care, or understand.

Seeking a feeling of certainty that will remain with you, you want more new tests performed or you want old tests repeated. You may spend endless hours seeking information or you may be afraid to even hear any casual mention of disease.

Problematic Body Focus 2: Symptoms Equal Debility

The second pattern that warns that you have gone too far in the direction of focusing on your body is when you let your bodily symptoms become the *sole* factor in deciding what you can and cannot do. It is especially easy to fall into this damaging body focus pattern after a serious illness or when you have chronic pain.

Remember that you, like everyone, have constantly changing physical sensations occurring in your body. It is your awareness of these background sensations and your conclusion about their meaning that fluctuates.

Sometimes you can come to believe that your physical symptoms mean that you are disabled, incapable, or unable to function. In other words, you conclude that symptoms equal debility.

You may jump to the conclusion that you can't do anything. You assume every physical sensation is the sign of disability or debility. You focus on your fatigue, pain, or other sensations to the exclusion of anything else.

You focus on symptoms when what you need to do is distract yourself, get busy, and ignore them. You may rest when you need to exert yourself and to be active despite symptoms.

The more you rest, the weaker muscles become. Weak muscles causes more fatigue and pain. Inactivity and lack of exercise worsen lymphedema due to lack of the muscle and joint actions that aid lymphatic drainage.

You may find yourself explaining to everyone that you cannot do things. When your health care professionals suggest that you increase your activities, you are sure they do not understand your condition. The most extreme form of this problematic body focus is sometimes called *somatization* or *somatoform disorder*.

Every sensation becomes a sign of catastrophe or disability. Your troubling sensations may seem always changing and unpredictable so you never know what you will feel or where in your body you will feel it.

The one thing that doesn't change is the conviction that you must always be on the alert and monitoring your body because something terrible is happening.

The Problem with Focusing on the Negative

An unchanging focus on the negative is damaging. This is true whether you focus on negative emotions, on negative interactions with others, or on negative changes in your body.

It is true that being aware of negatives helps us identify new or unresolved problems. But focusing on the negative is only a first, preliminary step in the process of finding a solution. It is not a solution itself.

Focusing on the negative does not solve anything. Focusing on the negative is not a good way to cope with problems.

In fact, focusing on the negative interferes with problem solving and coping. It uses mental and physical resources that could otherwise be redirected and used to cope and problem-solve. It narrows your focus to problems, not answers. And it drains you of hope.

Increased Body Focus in My Life Worksheet

Write your thoughts about what you have just read in Worksheet 8-1:

- List the ways you have increased your focus on your body in the first column.

- In the second column, record the positive or negative impact on your life of the increased body focus.

Here are some examples:

1. Since she developed lymphedema, Joan measures her arm according to the schedule her therapist gave her. She checks her body sensations briefly every morning and night and pays more attention to how her body feels if she has been particularly active. The impact on her life is that she spends some time each day on self-care, but she has less swelling, fewer infections and no hospitalizations, feels more confident, and is more and more active.

2. Evelyn has increased her focus on her body by measuring and checking several times every day regardless of the results and even though her therapist has told her she doesn't have to do this. She keeps her attention on her body and whenever she feels a new sensation, she wants to call her doctor and her lymphedema therapist. When she notices muscle soreness from exercise, she immediately stops what she is doing. She

Worksheet 8-1: Increased Body Focus In My Life

Impact On My Life and Lymphedema Care										
Specific Ways I Have Increased Focus On My Body										

does less and less even when her lymphedema is stable. Family members are getting tired of reassuring her and are becoming impatient.

Think about the information in this chapter. Review your answers and what you have learned.

Now, turn to Worksheet 14-2: **My Emotional Challenges** on page 201 and complete the line for "Increased body focus."

Resources

The Art of Getting Well: Maximizing Health and Well-Being When You Have a Chronic Illness by David Spero. Hunter House, 2002.

The Chronic Illness Workbook: Strategies and Solutions for Taking Back Your Life by Patricia Fennell. New Harbinger Publications, 2001.

Full Catastrophe Living: Using the Wisdom of Your Body and Mind to Face Stress, Pain, and Illness by John Kabat-Zinn, PhD. Dell Publishing, 1990.

Stop Worrying About Your Health: How to Quit Obsessing about your Symptoms and Feel Better Now by George Zgourides, PsyD. New Harbinger Publications, 2002.

Notes

1   If you are interested, one website is www.spiritabreast.com.

2   Kathryn Schmitz, PhD, MPH is the Principal Investigator of this planned study. See www.clinicaltrials.gov/ct/show/NCT00194363 for details.

Chapter 9

Self-Consciousness

Lymphedema can make a huge difference in how you look. It can affect what you can wear. It can affect how you feel about yourself.

Lymphedema is visible. You wonder whether others will notice. You wonder what they will think and how they will react.

> **66** I had done everything possible to look normal again…. But… I accidentally burned my arm on the stove. It became infected and the infection caused my arm to blow up like a balloon. It was grotesque.[1] **99**

Because people's reactions to us *are* influenced by our physical appearance, Chapter 10 is devoted to others' reactions and Chapter 18 covers communication skills for dealing with them. This chapter is devoted to you and your own reactions.

Normal Self-Consciousness

Feeling more self-conscious is a natural, and very common, response to secondary lymphedema because it changes the appearance of your body. Plus, whatever caused your lymphedema (for example, surgery, cancer, or burns) may also have changed your body's appearance. In one survey, 59% of cancer survivors reported that changes in appearance were a significant issue for them.[2]

The effect of primary lymphedema can vary depending on how old you are when it is diagnosed. On the one hand, the physical symptoms can increase the natural self-consciousness of adolescence. On the other hand, you may have had undiagnosed, untreated primary lymphedema for years. In this case, finally getting a diagnosis explains what's been happening in your body and gives you an opportunity to reduce its visible effects. Your feelings about your body may actually improve.

Normal Self-Consciousness and Sexuality

If you have an ongoing sexual relationship, you wonder how your partner will feel about the changes lymphedema causes. Will he or she still find you attractive? Will your body still be sexually arousing?

You may have trouble feeling sexually appealing. If you are not currently in a sexual relationship, you may worry about whether potential partners will be attracted to you.

Society gives us mixed messages about sexuality. Many people have conflicted feelings about sexuality and nudity. Take a minute to think about your feelings.

What were you taught about sexuality when you were younger? What positive sexual experiences have you had? What negative experiences have you had with sexuality? Summarize them here or write them down on another piece of paper:

_____

_____

Everything that happened in the past, good or bad, can continue to affect your sexuality. The effects of the past, and how to deal with them, are discussed in Chapter 12: Lessons from your Past.

When you develop lymphedema, it is perfectly normal to be more self-conscious during foreplay and sex. You may experience a temporary decrease in sexual desire or responsiveness, especially if you are also recovering from an accident or medical treatment.

Sexual arousal in the past may have occurred spontaneously, without much deliberate thought or effort. Now, you may need to work more deliberately to create and maintain arousal. These suggestions will help you overcome normal self-consciousness caused by lymphedema:

> ### *Coping Suggestions:*
>
> Don't panic, give up, or withdraw in response to temporary changes.
>
> Do work together with your partner. Talk about feelings. Explore together what is pleasurable to you both.
>
> Share non-sexual, pleasurable touching.
>
> You may want to spend more time on foreplay.
>
> Take an active role in building and sustaining your arousal by deliberately focusing on pleasurable physical sensations during foreplay and sex.
>
> Actively encourage pleasure by focusing on memories or images that are sexually arousing. Some people find that romantic or erotic novels, movies, or pictures are an effective way to stimulate arousal.
>
> Your goal is to share pleasure.

You and Your Body

Ideally, self-consciousness decreases over time. You accept your body as it is and take steps to keep it healthy and functioning to the best of its ability. You see your body as heroically doing its best and as deserving your support, your guidance, and your respect.

Recollect what you learned in Chapter 1 about how your body interacts with your mind, with your actions, with your emotions, and with your thoughts. Because we live this life embodied in a physical frame, we often think of our bodies and our selves as being one and the same.

When we look in a mirror, we say that we see ourselves. When what we see has changed, it is a challenge to us. It is normal to go through a temporary period of increased self-consciousness that lessens over time.

Your challenge is to successfully incorporate lymphedema-related physical changes into your view of yourself. You want the increase in painful self-consciousness to be temporary. You do not want to live with a sense of shame or guilt.

You want to develop a positive view of yourself and a positive relationship with your body.

Your Relationship with Your Body

The next three worksheets let you explore your relationship with your body. People think about and process things in different ways. Some people are very visual. They may think and react using symbols or images. Others are more feeling-oriented. Others are more verbal. According to your preferences, use some or all of the exercises in the next three worksheets (9-1, 9-2, and 9-3) to explore your relationship with your body.

Your Feelings About Your Body

Pick an image that symbolically represents your body. It can be an animal, a plant, or some living being. It can be something from nature, something man-made, or something completely imagined. It can be a cartoon character. It could just be how you picture your body in your mind and what parts of your body you emphasize. Write down (or sketch) the images that come into your mind in the left column of Worksheet 9-1

Now, as you think about each image, write down your feelings in the right hand column.

Reflect on what you learned in this exercise. It is natural to feel a mixture of emotions, positive and negative.

What emotions are strongest? _____

Which emotion(s) do you feel most often? _____

Your goal is to decrease the negative feelings and increase your positive feelings toward your body.

Worksheet 9-1: My Body and Me—Images and Feelings

My Feelings	The Image(s) That Represent My Body

Negative Feelings

Which emotion(s) cause you the most distress or interfere with your lymphedema care or your overall functioning, happiness, or quality of life?

_____

- **If anger and/or resentment are your primary feelings**, reread Chapter 4: Anger and Resentment. Work to discover what feelings are behind your anger and what feelings are maintaining it.

- **If you are feeling overwhelmed, hopeless, or unable to move on beyond grief**, turn to Chapter 2: Feeling Overwhelmed, Chapter 3: Sadness and Grieving, and Chapter 11: Searching for Meaning.

- **If your main emotion is fear**, think about what you fear and how this fear manifests itself in your thoughts and actions. Review Chapters 5 through 8 and reread the parts that apply to you.

- **If your main emotion is guilt or self-blame**, complete this chapter and then turn to Chapter 11: Searching for Meaning.

- **If you are aware of feelings of shame, embarrassment, disgust, or revulsion**, read this chapter very closely.

Positive Feelings

Review the body images you identified in Worksheet 9-1 for positive feelings. Think about your body:

- Do you feel gratitude toward your body for what it has allowed you to do and experience in the past? Do you feel gratitude for what your body allows you to do now (even though changed or limited by lymphedema)?

- Do you feel admiration or respect for your body's efforts to cope with the lymphedema as best it can?

- Do you feel loving care toward your body? Do you feel sympathy or concern for its struggles?

- Do you feel a sense of commitment to your body? Do you feel a partnership with it in meeting the challenges of lymphedema?

If you didn't have any positive feelings, begin to think about how you would like to feel toward your body. You will explore this more in Worksheet 9-2: My Body and Me—Dialogue.

Your Thoughts about Your Body

Let's explore another aspect of your relationship to your body that will affect how self-conscious you will feel—your thoughts. What we say to ourselves has an enormous impact on our feelings.

What are you saying to yourself about your body? If you imagine yourself talking to your body, what are you saying to it or about it? Write the words in the left hand column of the worksheet.

If your body could talk to you, what would it say in reply? Write your body's reply in the right column.

Here is an example:

What I Say To My Body Or About My Body	What My Body Would Say If It Could Speak
You're so ugly because of lymphedema. I can't stand you! You're big and heavy and swollen and uncomfortable. I hate you!	*Do you think I like being this way? I didn't choose this any more than you did. You hating and berating me doesn't help. If my lymph system could move the lymph, it would.*
I do hate lymphedema but I'll work with you. I'll look for early warning signs of flare-ups or infection and I'll try to protect you.	*Thank you. Things are so much better when you watch out for me and protect me. Whatever I can do on my own, I will.*

Reread what you wrote. How do you feel about your relationship with your body? Do you like the relationship you have with your body?

Do you like the things you are saying and thinking? Are you saying things that make you feel more accepting?

Or are your words making you feel more ashamed, more disgusted, or more distressed?

Improving Your Relationship with Your Body

This exercise will help you explore changes that you would like to make in your relationship with your body:

- Review what you wrote in Worksheet 9-1 on page 103.

- In the top part of Worksheet 9-3, write images you would like to represent your body.

- Then, write the feelings you want to have toward your body.

- Now review what you wrote in Worksheet 9-2 on page 107.

- Write the kinds of things you would like to say to and about your body.

- Now write what you would like your body to say to you if it could speak.

Mary's Story

I'm an artist and after my lymphedema diagnosis, I keep seeing my body like it was a broken, useless machine on the junk heap. Every time that picture came into my mind, I felt hopeless and worthless. I heard myself thinking and saying, *"Nothing works. I can't trust on my body any more. I can't rely on it. I hate my body."* And it was like my body was saying, *"I'm a lost cause. You'll never be able to do anything you enjoy again. No one will love you. Your life is ruined."*

Luckily, the support of my friends and family got me through. I found a terrific lymphedema therapist. I picked myself up by my bootstraps and decided that life had to go on. I learned about lymphedema. I do my treatments and follow my self-management routine. I've had some rough times but I'm doing a lot better now.

My image of my body has really changed. The machine may be battered and mended, but it is working again. When I picture that I feel sympathy and respect. I feel like I re-established a caring relationship with my body. I think, *"You're doing your best and I can and will help you. Together we will make a life. Life goes on."* If my body could talk, I think it would say, *"You're doing a good job of taking care of me and I appreciate it. You can trust me to do my very best to take good care of you. After all, we're in this together."*

Worksheet 9-2: My Body and Me—Dialogue

What My Body Would Say If It Could Speak											
What I Say To My Body Or About My Body											

Reducing Normal Self-Consciousness

Reflect on what you have learned so far. You may have a positive relationship with your body or you may be seeing positive changes and decreasing self-consciousness.

If this is the case, congratulate yourself. Ask yourself:

*   What have I done that has made these positive changes possible?

    _____

*   What has helped reduce uncomfortable self-consciousness and protect a positive relationship with my body?

    _____

*   Can I use what I have learned to further improve this relationship?

    _____

If these worksheets highlighted problem areas in your relationship with your body, then congratulate yourself on having the honesty and courage to complete them. The first step toward increased self-acceptance is identifying problem areas.

The changes of lymphedema can undermine self-esteem and self-confidence. These suggestions can counter that process:

Coping Suggestions:

Think about everything that makes you uniquely you.

List what makes you the person you are, separate from your body. You could include your values, your religious/spiritual/philosophical beliefs, your relationships, your personality traits, etc., etc.

Reread it daily. Add to it as more things come to mind.

Deliberately remind yourself: "I am more than my physical body. I am not my lymphedema." Act on these words.

Worksheet 9-2: My Body and Me—A Changed Relationship

The image(s) I would *like* to symbolize my body are:	The feelings I would *like* to have toward my body and its image(s) are:	What I would *like* to say to and about my body:	What I would *like* to have my body say to me if it could speak:

A changed awareness of your body is inevitable with lymphedema. Increased self-consciousness is normal.

Ongoing, intense self-consciousness that interferes with your life or happiness is not inevitable. The rest of this chapter explores the more troublesome forms of self-consciousness in more depth.

Problematic Self-Consciousness

Some degree of self-consciousness and concern about others' reactions is natural when you have a condition that affects your appearance. Coming to terms with visible physical changes and others' reactions is challenging.

At best, such a challenge forces upon us the opportunity to grow. We think about what really defines us. We increase awareness of our core values.

At worst, this challenge amplifies any pre-existing issues related to your body or your self-worth. You may find yourself ashamed, embarrassed, and hiding. Feelings of disgust or revulsion may develop or increase.

Risk Factors for Problematic Self-Consciousness

If you were shy or self-conscious before the lymphedema, you may now want to crawl into a shell. Previous self-consciousness is contributing to a problematic reaction.

If before lymphedema, you defined yourself and your self-worth on the basis of your physical attractiveness, lymphedema changes may seem unacceptable and intolerable. You may feel that you have lost your identity or self-image.

If you respond to discomfort by avoiding other people, self-consciousness will be more difficult to handle. It will also be less likely to resolve on its own over time.

If you generally tend to focus on the negative aspects of any situation, problematic self-consciousness is more likely. Focusing on negative physical changes can cause you to lose sight of everything else that defines you as a unique and complex person of interest, capability, and worth. You may lose all perspective on how your body looks to others.

Warning Signs

Are you doing things differently out of self-consciousness? Check those that apply to you:

☐ **Are you refusing physical contact with your partner?** Are you avoiding talking about your feelings or your partner's feeling? Are you giving up and not trying ways to regain a rewarding sexual life?

☐ **Are you refusing to go out to places, see friends, and participate in activities?** Are you refusing to wear clothes you want to wear that are comfortable, attractive, and non-binding solely because they feel too revealing of your lymphedema to others?

☐ **Are you refusing to be in situations where you are among strangers?** Are you refusing to talk, go on dates, or initiate or respond to sexual overtures? Are you are refusing to make eye contact with others for fear of seeing a negative reaction?

Immediately after first being diagnosed, you may temporarily withdraw from others. This is understandable. As you adjust to living with lymphedema, you resume involvement with people.

Problems occur when such withdrawal actions are not temporary. If you checked any of the boxes above, ask yourself, *"Am I responding to my concerns by using avoidance? Am I letting my self-consciousness restrict my life?"*

The Problem with Avoidance

Why *not* use avoidance in dealing with self-consciousness? It seems so easy and tempting. People who care about you may even encourage you to avoid, advising you not to make yourself uncomfortable.

Research findings in this area are consistent, strong, and clear.[3] Hiding, withdrawing, or avoiding actually maintains your negative feelings about your body.

Avoiding leaves you convinced that your worst fears are true—because you never test them out. It may *feel* safer, but it takes away the opportunity to discover when your fears are distorted, exaggerated, or just not true.

If there are people who don't notice or aren't bothered by your lymphedema, you want to find them. The alternative is to stay huddled and withdrawn, closeted with your fears, shame, or disgust.

Being restricted by self-concerns can be like living in a dark cave or a cramped jail cell. You want to make free choices about what you do or don't do. When self-consciousness dictates or restricts your actions, you are not free.

Finally, avoiding removes opportunities to develop skills you can use to cope with the problems of self-consciousness or with others' responses. You lose the chance to become stronger and more self-assured. You give up important longer-term benefits in order to avoid short-term emotional discomfort.

Let's look at the uncomfortable emotions that can lead you to restrict your life:

- Embarrassment, anxiety, and worry or

- Disgust, revulsion, and shame.

Problematic Self-Consciousness 1: Embarrassment, Anxiety, Worry

Sometimes the emotions underlying our self-consciousness are those of embarrassment, anxiety, and/or worry.

Check the items that apply to you. Do you:

☐ Only feel comfortable when you are alone or with people with whom you feel safe?

☐ Worry about embarrassing yourself in social situations? Expect, or fear, that others will judge or criticize you in social situations?

☐ Avoid, or endure with distress, situations such as parties, making conversation, speaking up in class or at work?

☐ Worry that you anxiety will interfere with your performance?

☐ Continue to be predictably anxious in these situations?

☐ Think that your fear might be out of proportion to the actual risk, at least sometimes?

If you checked one or more of the boxes above, you may have a problem that is anxiety-based called *social anxiety disorder* or *social phobia*.

You may notice problems in all situations involving other people or just some situations. These feelings may have troubled you most of your life or they may have started since you developed lymphedema or experienced the physical changes that lead to lymphedema.

The tools and skills in Section IV may give you what you need to overcome this challenge. See also **Resources** for Social Anxiety at the end of this chapter.

If these feelings continue to trouble you, find a professional who treats social anxiety. Specific psychotherapy treatments and medications can help. Cognitive-behavioral therapy, where you actively challenge your thinking and confront your fears, is effective for social anxiety.

What if the emotion underlying your painful self-consciousness is *not* anxiety?

Problematic Self-Consciousness 2: Disgust, Revulsion, Shame

Most of us are at least somewhat dissatisfied with some aspect of our physical appearance.[4] After all, look at the images and the messages that surround us on television, in magazines, and in the movies.

Media and advertisements continually tell us that we could and should be physically perfect. We are bombarded by unreal images of perfection.

Models and stars are made up by professional make-up artists. They have their hair and clothes arranged by professional stylists. They are photographed by professional photographers who use camera filters and computer programs to make create perfect images that are not real.

Even these most beautiful people in the world at the height of their physical beauty don't look as good as their pictures!

But no one talks about that truth. That would not sell products. Instead the messages are constantly sent that:

- Physical perfection is possible and necessary.

- You have to be perfect to be sexually appealing, loved, happy, or successful.

Believing these distorted media messages, makes it very hard to accept the physical changes of lymphedema and still feel good about yourself.

Review your answers to the three **My Body And Me** Worksheets on pages 103, 107, and 109, that you completed earlier.

- Do you struggle with disgust, revulsion, and/or shame?

- Do you feel this way about your body occasionally, frequently, or constantly?

- Do you have the ability to talk back to these feelings, to challenge them, and to replace them with other thoughts?

- Do you spend much of your time preoccupied with such thoughts or taking actions based on them?

People who are demanding perfectionists are very likely to feel shame. People who are depressed are very likely to think negative thoughts about their appearance.

But it works the other way as well. The more critical you are of your body, the more likely you are to feel depressed.

Body Dysmorphic Disorder

Sometimes these thoughts and feelings reach such intensity that the problem is what is known as *body dysmorphic disorder*. Some of the signs of body dysmorphic disorder are that you:

☐ Are intensely distressed by your physical imperfection. You think things such as, *"I am grotesque. I am a monster. I look disgusting. I am deformed. Other people must be revolted by me."*

☐ Believe that others experience the same emotional reaction to your body's imperfections that you do, or they would if you didn't hide or disguise the imperfections.

☐ Disbelieve others when they say that they are not revolted or disgusted by your physical appearance or that your body doesn't look as bad as you think.

☐ Are preoccupied with thoughts of how horrific your body is.

☐ Are preoccupied with ways to disguise or minimize your physical imperfections.

If you marked most or all of the boxes above, read the self-help workbooks on Body Image in the **Resources** section at the end of this chapter. Consider getting professional help for psychotherapy and/or medication that may help you challenge and change these distressing and destructive thoughts and actions.

The Benefits of Challenging Problematic Self-Consciousness

As you can see, problematic self-consciousness involves:

• Negative conclusions about your body

• Negative assumptions about the reactions of others to you

• Discounting or disbelieving any evidence that your negative conclusions may be wrong or exaggerated

• Focusing on your imperfections and often avoiding, hiding, minimizing, or trying to disguise them.

This is a self-perpetuating cycle. You don't have to go along with it. It will not change on its own, but you can fight back and work to regain more comfort and acceptance regardless of your appearance.

> ## *Coping Suggestions:*
>
> Look at the consequences of thinking and acting in this way. If you don't like the results, try the experiment of deliberately changing.
>
> Take a risk. Remind yourself: *"Just because I think something is true or believe it is true, does not mean it is true".*
>
> Encourage yourself to challenge the negative thoughts. Deliberately replace them with thoughts that give you permission to be happy and active despite your imperfections.
>
> Accept physical imperfection. But then refuse to let it alone dictate what you do.
>
> Don't avoid people, places, things, or activities just because you aren't perfect.
>
> Don't withdraw from life because of lymphedema.

Taking this approach to visible body changes is hard, especially at first. But persevere. By vigorously challenging your thoughts and changing your actions, research shows that you can gain positive long-term results:[5]

- Self-image and self-esteem increase regardless of your appearance.

- You become more confident.

- You experience less distress.

- Your interpersonal skills improve.

- You have more satisfying interactions with others.

Changing your relationship with your body and decreasing painful self-consciousness may take time. Give yourself this time. See the **Resources** listed below and use ideas and skills from other chapters.

The website www.changingfaces.org.uk may help you with ideas and inspiration. It was designed by and for people with visible physical changes and emphasizes overcoming self-consciousness.

Portions of Chapter 13: Current Life Stresses may be relevant. Ideas from the earlier chapters may apply. Section IV: Tools for Change presents a comprehensive toolbox of skills for change.

Self-Consciousness and Its Impact on Your Life

Think about your answers to the questions and Worksheets in this chapter. Review your answers and what you have learned about the impact of self-consciousness on your life.

Now, turn to Worksheet 14-2: **My Emotional Challenges** on page 201 and complete the line for "Self-Consciousness".

Resources

Social Anxiety Resources

Dying of Embarrassment: Help for Social Anxiety and Phobia by Barbara Markway, PhD, Cheryl Carmin, PhD, C. Alec Pollard, PhD, and Teresa Flynn, PhD. New Harbinger Publications, 1992.

The Shyness and Social Anxiety Workbook: Proven Techniques for Overcoming Your Fears by Martin Antony, PhD and Richard Swinson, MD. New Harbinger Publications, 2000.

Body Image Resources

The Body Image Workbook: An 8-step Program for Learning to Like Your Looks by Thomas F. Cash, PhD. New Harbinger, 1997.

The BDD Workbook: Overcome Body Dysmorphic Disorder and End Body Image Obsessions by James Claiborn, PhD and Cherry Pedrick, RN. New Harbinger Publications, 2002.

Changing Faces web site www.changingfaces.org.uk

Notes

1   **Winning the Race** by Nancy Brinker and Chriss Winston. Tapestry Press, 2001. p. 63.

2   **LIVESTRONG Poll Fact Sheet** by the Lance Armstrong Foundation, November 30, 2004.

3   **The Body Image Workbook: An 8-step Program for Learning to Like Your Looks** by Thomas F. Cash, PhD. New Harbinger, 1997.

4   **The Body Image Workbook: An 8-step Program for Learning to Like Your Looks** by Thomas F. Cash, PhD. New Harbinger, 1997.

5   **The Body Image Workbook: An 8-step Program for Learning to Like Your Looks** by Thomas F. Cash, PhD. New Harbinger, 1997.

Chapter **10:**

Handling Others' Reactions

What reactions to your lymphedema can you expect from other people? How can you deal with these reactions? Others' reactions can be negative, positive, or mixed. Often they will experience different emotions at different times. Some people won't even notice anything at all.

As You Read This Chapter

As you read this chapter, think about how other people react to your lymphedema. Think about how you respond. And, finally, consider the impact on your life.

Use what you learn to complete Worksheet 10-1: The Impact of Others' Reactions on My Life on page 133. You may want to work on it as you read along.

Later in this book, Chapter 18 provides specific communication skills to help you deal with other people and their reactions to you and your lymphedema. If you are having difficulties with a healthcare professional, read the section devoted to dealing with healthcare providers, starting on page 308.

Positive Reactions from Others

Take a moment and recall positive reactions you have encountered from others. Sometimes we remember the negative and forget the positive, so focus on those positive memories right now.

A positive reaction could be someone unobtrusively helping you. It could be words of praise, encouragement and support. It could be a quick hug from a friend, or a coworker who shows genuine interest and treats you as the whole person you are. It could be someone letting you know that they respect and admire you or that how you deal with your lymphedema inspires them or has helped others.

When you get positive reactions from others, notice them. Show your appreciation. Let others know how those positive reactions make you feel.

React in ways that make such positive reactions more likely. Smile. Thank them. Compliment them. Work to increase the number of positive reactions.

Identify those people who help you reach your emotional and physical goals. You want to strengthen these important relationships in your life. Spend more time with those people.

Curiosity from Others

You can anticipate that people will be curious about your swelling, bandages, or compression garment. What you say and how much detailed information you share will depend on your preference and your relationship to the person asking.

When you know the person asking questions, you'll probably give a brief, honest explanation. Think ahead about the amount and type of information you want to share depending on the circumstance and the closeness of your relationship with the other person.

Some people like the idea of a lymphedema information card that they can hand out. LymphNotes.com has developed a card the size of a standard business card that provides basic information about lymphedema; send an e-mail to cards@LymphNotes.com for a free copy.

Other people with lymphedema find it easier to give a simple, routine response to strangers' questions. Here are some examples: *"I have a swelling problem." "Thank you for your concern. It's nothing to worry about."*

Some people with lymphedema make a game of creating outrageous answers when responding to strangers. For example, Barbara Abercrombie writes, *"I vary my routine with curious strangers; sometimes I tell them it was a skydiving accident, sometimes it happened when I was surfing. I've become the Walter Mitty of risky sports."*[1]

What to say is your personal decision. The amount and type of information you share is up to you.

Negative Reactions from Others

You are likely to have already encountered negative reactions from others. I hope the ideas and suggestions here will both reduce any distress caused by these reactions and increase your confidence in your ability to handle them.

It helps if you can understand and expect some of the frequent negative reactions. Coping with a negative reaction is easier when you have planned in advance and are not taken by surprise.

You want to resolve or avoid negative interactions when you can. When this is not possible, you want to decrease them and cope with them when they do occur.

You want to ensure that other people's reactions do not interfere with your taking care of yourself, physically and emotionally. You want to protect your relationships from damage.

Family

The most important "others" in your life are often family members. Very close friends may be like family. The ideas in this section can apply to them as well. Identify who is "family" to you:

- Who lives with you? _____

- Who is close to you physically? _____

- Who is close to you emotionally? _____

Most people have never heard of lymphedema. Your family may have no idea what is involved or how to help.

Talk with family members openly about how you feel and what you need. Listen to them about how they feel and what they need.

Challenge as an Opportunity

When one partner in a relationship develops a chronic condition, the relationship changes In one survey of cancer survivors, about half (54%) of the respondents reported problems in their relationships with friends and family and said that they had noticed more emotional distance between them and important people in their lives.[2] But this is not inevitable. Other research shows that families can be very resilient.[3]

You can influence your family's reactions. If you are overwhelmed and don't care for your body, the result can be worsening symptoms or medical crises. As a result, your family's negative reactions can be more frequent and more severe.

The opposite is true. The more you use the tools in this book to help you cope well, emotionally and physically, the more you increase the chances that your family members will cope well.

Family members *can* successfully meet the challenges of chronic illness and the rewards are substantial. Relationships can become deeper, closer, more intimate, more satisfying, and happier. Psychological growth can result from facing the crisis of disease.[4]

Successfully working through the emotional and practical problems posed by lymphedema leads to a deeper sense of respect, confidence, and trust.

Your Partner's Reactions

What normal reactions can you expect? Your partner is likely to experience several of the same emotional challenges that you face.

What can you do? Share this book. Share some of the ideas and techniques you learn. Communicate. Listen. Your partner may communicate differently than you do.

Take into account differences in communication style and coping. Some people cope by talking about issues over and over again, while others need time alone. Some are more feeling-oriented; others focus more on facts and actions. See Chapter 18 for specific communications skills.

You or your partner may experience a temporary decrease in sexual desire or responsiveness. If this occurs, review the information relating to sexuality in Chapter 9: Self-Consciousness.

Children's Reactions

Children see the world in terms of themselves. This is normal and healthy. When a parent is ill, children often worry:

- Did I cause it? Did I hurt my parent in some way? Is this my fault?
- Is it a punishment?
- Will it hurt mommy or daddy if I touch or hug her/him?
- Can I catch it? Will other family members get sick?
- Will my parent die?
- Who will take care of me?

If it is a child or teenager who has lymphedema, the other siblings will have the questions listed above. They may have other questions as well:

- Did it happen because of something I said or did or wished?
- Could I accidentally hurt them? Are they going to die?
- Do they get special treatment because our parents love them best?
- Am I unimportant? Am I second best?
- Can I ask for what I want and say what I feel?

Use language the children can understand and that is appropriate to their ages and their personalities. You may want to state important information simply and repeat it often at first. These communication skills are discussed in greater detail in Chapter 23: For Parents of Children with Lymphedema.

Negative Reactions

Some reactions may be negative, even from your loving family. They may be confused, frightened or angry.

Confusion, Lack of Knowledge, Misinformation

Your family and others who care for you may experience some of the same emotional reactions that you do. Or, because each person is different, they may have trouble understanding how you feel.

The more you can listen to their feelings, the more likely they are to be able to listen to yours. Reading some or all of the chapters in this book should also be helpful.

Those who care about you may not know how to help you practically, for example, by assisting with bandaging. They may not understand what you need emotionally. They may wonder why you can't do things you used to do. They may feel confused and bewildered.

They may give you bad advice while trying to be helpful because they don't understand about lymphedema. You need to educate yourself. Then you can help to educate them.

Think about how they learn. Some people learn best by reading, others by talking. Some people only understand after they see something or do it for themselves. The book, **Living Well With Lymphedema**, gives a lot of practical information and advice with descriptions and pictures.

Be prepared to explain more than once. Be patient as you remind them of what has changed. Remember that they are dealing with their own emotional challenges. In fact, they may benefit by having a personal copy of this book so they can read the chapters for family members plus whatever other chapters will be most useful.

Sometimes it helps to have someone else explain about lymphedema and how family can help. Most lymphedema therapists are delighted to have a family member accompany you to a treatment session, or even have a private session alone, so that the therapist can answer questions and demonstrate lymphedema treatment.

Guide them to reliable sources of trustworthy information. (See **Resources** at the end of this chapter for books and web sites.) The more everyone knows, the more effectively you all can work together to understand and manage lymphedema.

Show appreciation for helpful acts—even the small ones. Step by step, you and your family can learn, adjust, and make the changes that let you live a life that is different than before lymphedema, but that is healthy, happy, and full.

Fear, Anxiety, Worry

It's scary to have someone you love be diagnosed with lymphedema. People respond to fear in different ways.

Some people will worry that you are fragile and will respond by becoming overprotective. They may take over tasks that you can and should do yourself. Others worry that you are not taking good care of yourself. Out of concern, they become watchful and start to nag or give orders.

Sometimes others pull away emotionally. They may fear that they can't meet your needs. They may worry that you will no longer be able to take care of them. They may worry that you will die and so they distance themselves because the thought of losing you hurts. Your lymphedema may trigger within them a sense of their own vulnerability and mortality.

Remind yourself that fear is uncomfortable for them. They are probably responding to it the best way they know. Address their underlying concerns. If they believe there is less to be worried and anxious about, then they'll be more able to change their actions.

Pity

Pity is feeling sorry for someone. This is different from empathy, which is understanding what the other person is going through.

You want people to understand your struggles and to support you. You don't want them to see you as a helpless victim. Sometimes family members give more help than you want; sometimes they give less help than you need.

You are challenged, but you are not helpless. Learn how to help yourself. Make sure you are doing your part. Show them what you can do. Teach them how to help you take care of yourself.

Anger, Impatience

Any of the feelings above can result in someone feeling angry, irritable, or impatient. People frequently become angry or impatient if they feel frightened, hurt, or helpless. Other triggers for anger are feeling threatened or believing that something is wrong or unfair.

Encourage the other person to talk about the underlying feelings beneath the anger. Those feelings could be any of the feelings discussed so far.

If your family member is often angry:

- Review Chapter 4: Anger and Resentment.
- Use the communication skills in Chapter 18.

If your family member gets physically abusive when angry, this may be a Red Flag:

- Skip ahead to Chapter 13 and read the Red Flag warning signs .
- If any of them apply, read the entire section on in Chapter 13 on "Problematic Interpersonal Stresses."

Nobody's Perfect

Just like you, your family members can face emotional challenges in dealing with lymphedema. They may have limits on their time, their skill, their knowledge and education, or their energy.

Your lymphedema may activate issues from the other person's past. For example:

- Some people are able to meet another person's practical needs, but have trouble responding to their emotional needs.

- Others may have particular difficulty dealing with illness, permitting appropriate dependence, or accepting changes in appearance, because of personal past experiences, childhood, values, or personality. They may tend to be self-conscious or pessimistic and too easily dwell only on the negative facts about lymphedema.

- They may feel guilty about being healthy, about needing help from you, or not being able to take care of you the way they think they should. They may feel guilty about having negative emotions at all – even though such feelings are normal reactions.

Try to understand each other. Talk. Face and solve the problems of lymphedema together rather than letting lymphedema divide you.

Accept that everyone has limits. If you can't get what you need from one person, turn to another.

Seek a balance in your life together that works for both you and your partner. Dealing with lymphedema is important, but there is more to life than self-management. Look for things to enjoy together. Have fun. Enjoy.

Positive Reactions

Your family may also have positive reactions leading to collaboration, respect, and hope.

Collaboration

Some family members may be able to work with you. Some may provide practical support; others, emotional support. Deeper, honest, and respectful communication can lead to greater understanding and real empathy for one another. Effective teamwork and increased emotional closeness may result.

Respect, Pride, Confidence

Your family may develop pride and respect for you as they see you handling your lymphedema skillfully. They too may develop more independence and more confidence as they learn how to cope along with you.

Family and close friends may show you that they still accept, care for, and value you as you are. They may be a source of support and praise to help you put forth the effort to deal well with your lymphedema. You may be able to confidently turn to them and rely on them.

Hope

Sometimes family members, or close friends, can be your own personal cheerleading team. They may believe in you and what you can achieve—even before you do. They may be able to emphasize the positive, even while acknowledging the negative.

Encourage your family—and yourself—to be realistically optimistic whenever possible. Lymphedema can improve. Treatment can help. Flare-ups can resolve. Progress in treatment is possible.

Notice any of the above positive reactions. Appreciate and foster them.

Healthcare Professionals

On the positive side, your healthcare providers may be caring, interested, and encouraging. They may be eager to teach what they know and eager to learn from you and expand their knowledge. The may work collaboratively with you in a mutually respectful partnership.

On the negative side, your caregivers may seem arrogant, uninterested, uninformed, unhelpful, and/or uncaring. They may downplay the seriousness of the condition (*"It's just a little swelling."*) They may know little about treatment procedures and resources and seem uninterested in learning anything from you.

If you want to educate your care provider about lymphedema, be aware that some sources of information are considered far more credible than others:

- Articles published in professional journals are usually far more convincing than articles from newspapers or general magazines.

- Information that is based on research and that comes from books written by other professionals who cite research is more convincing than information obtained from the Internet.

- Hard evidence is more convincing than stories. For example, measurements of your body area before and after compression and manual lymph drainage is more compelling than just saying, *"I think it helps."*

Coping Suggestions:

Consider recommending specific books or websites. Be willing to briefly explain why those sources of information are reliable. See Chapter 6 for tips on evaluating information sources.

Make it fast and easy for the other person to get the information you want them to have. Like you, they have many competing demands.

Read Chapter 18: Communication Skills. The points above are explained in more detail in the section devoted to communicating with healthcare professionals. Use the communication skills taught throughout the chapter.

Bosses, Coworkers, Friends, and Acquaintances

What about people outside the family? What emotions can you expect them to feel?

They may feel uncomfortable and not know what to do. Be prepared to deal with some awkwardness. Humans can react to emotional discomfort or uncertainty in a number of unhelpful ways.

When people don't know what to do, they become anxious and uncomfortable. They don't know how to handle their discomfort and, therefore, don't act naturally. As a result, they often do or say tactless things.

You may worry that you will not be hired or promoted and there may be some basis for this concern. Research *has* shown that people with visibly disfiguring conditions tend to be seen as less competent.

On the other hand, you have more power than you may think. The same research studies found that how you present yourself with others can *counteract* the negative effect of visible disfigurement.[5] See Chapter 18 Communications Skills resources.

Your boss and coworkers will have many worries and may not deal with these concerns skillfully or tactfully. They may fear that you will become ill and disabled. They may wonder whether lymphedema is contagious—which, of course, it is not.

If your boss fears you have a chronic medical condition that will cost the company money, you may worry that your boss will fire you. If this is a concern, get as many facts as possible.

If possible, talk to your boss about any concerns he or she may have. Consider talking to your union or consulting an attorney who specializes in this area of law. You may need to become familiar with relevant employment laws.

If your coworkers and acquaintances see visible signs of lymphedema such as swelling, bandages or compression garments, they may be uncomfortable and avoid you—or they may want all the gory details. Discomfort and ignorance can lead to misinformation, rumors, or misunderstandings.

Some people may not understand why you need accommodation or how to accommodate you. They may expect too much and feel impatient or resentful.

Others may feel pity. They may see you as "disabled" rather than as a talented, knowledgeable person who simply needs some physical assistance. These people may try to give you more help than you want or need. They may foster a destructive sense that you are helpless. Do not fall into this trap.

Coping Suggestions:

Before you return to work or go for an interview, decide whether you want to say anything about your lymphedema. How much detail you give will vary from person to person.

Decide ahead of time what you are comfortable saying. Address people's fears in terms that they can understand.

Practice what you want to say over and over. Rehearse it aloud until you say it comfortably, easily, and confidently.

Use the communication skills in Chapter 18 to defuse feelings.

Educate others about lymphedema as appropriate, but don't let lymphedema define who you are.

Emphasize your talents and worth by your words and your actions.

Strangers

What about strangers who know nothing about your lymphedema? What do you do when people stare? How do you respond to questions? These questions highlight an important issue.

Negative Reactions

Perhaps, before you developed lymphedema, you were able to be anonymous in a crowd and look like everyone else. It can be comforting to blend in and not draw attention if you don't want it.

If your lymphedema is visible, you may have lost this ability. People may ask you questions. They may stare. You may encounter curiosity or outright rudeness. You may experience prejudice, rejection, or avoidance.

Strangers may avoid eye contact with you or they may stare. They may avoid talking with you at all or they may ask personal questions.

Coping Suggestions:

Decide in advance what you feel comfortable telling strangers.

Practice until you are comfortable saying it.

Positive Reactions

Strangers may also offer sympathy and support. They may respect your privacy. They may tactfully offer appropriate assistance when needed.

Neutral Reactions

It is also, of course, possible that strangers may not even notice the physical effects of lymphedema. These effects may seem glaringly obvious to you; but that is because you are focused on them.

Remember, other people are usually much more focused on themselves than they are on anyone else. They have their own lives, their own concerns, and their own troubles and tragedies.

You Have Power

Others do respond to our appearance. But, first impressions and negative reactions can be changed. Understanding that negative reactions can occur and preparing your response makes sense.

Research clearly shows we can counteract the effect of our appearance. Our manner of interacting with others, our comfort level, and our actions strongly influence other people. In fact, these variables outweigh the effect of appearance.

When others seem uncomfortable in your presence, they may well be responding more to your actions than to your appearance.

The research in this area is consistent and encouraging. People with a number of visibly disfiguring conditions have been studied and taught to change how they act around other people. Their changed behavior changed the way others reacted to them.

The specific techniques listed in the Coping Suggestions have been proven to powerfully impact others' reactions and impressions.

> ### *Coping Suggestions:*
> Keep your head up.
>
> Deliberately make eye contact.
>
> Smile often. Nod frequently.
>
> Use a confident, but friendly tone of voice.
>
> Hold your body in a relaxed, friendly, and confident manner.
>
> Rehearse and practice these actions until you do them skillfully.

If you are already these things, applaud yourself. If these actions are new for you, you may see changes in how you feel about yourself as you change your behavior. Our feelings are far more strongly affected by what we say to ourselves and how we behave than by how we look.

If you find this hard to believe, look at the research. How uncomfortable we feel about our bodies and in social situations has very little to do with how much actual disfigurement we have.[6]

This may be surprising to you. It is worth repeating because it opens the door to hope and action. Your level of disfigurement does not control your level of comfort.

You have more power than you think. Use it. That's the purpose of this book.

The Impact of Others' Reactions on Your Life

Think about others' reactions and how they impact you:

- List specific people or groups of people under Who in the first column of worksheet 10-1.

- Summarize their reactions in the second column.

- Summarize how you are responding currently in the third column.

- Evaluate the impact this has on you in the fourth column.

Review your answers to the Worksheet:

- Do you like the way you are behaving toward others? _____

Worksheet 10-1: The Impact of Others' Reactions On My Life

Who?	Their Reactions	My Response	Impact On My Life

- Is there anything in your action that you want to change? _____
- What is the impact on your emotional well-being, on your lymph-edema self-management, and on your quality of life? _____

Now, turn to Worksheet 14-2: **My Emotional Challenges** on page 201 and complete the line for "Others' reactions."

Resources

Lymphedema Information

Living Well With Lymphedema by Ann Ehrlich, Alma Vinjé-Harrewijn, PT, CLT and Elizabeth McMahon, PhD Lymph Notes, 2005.

Lymphedema: A Breast Cancer Patient's Guide To Prevention And Healing by Jeannie Burt and Gwen White. Publishers Group West, 1999.

Coping With Lymphedema by Joan Swirsky and Dianne Nannery. Avery Publishing Group, 1998.

www.LymphNotes.com an online resource and support group for persons with lymphedema and their family members and for lymphedema thera-pists. It also provides information about lymphedema, treatment resources, and support groups.

www.lymphnet.org website of the National Lymphedema Network, a nonprofit organization providing information about lymphedema, treat-ment resources, and support groups.

General Communication Skills

Why Marriages Succeed Or Fail: And How You Can Make Yours Last by John Gottman. Simon & Schuster, 1995.

The Relationship Cure: A 5 Step Guide to Strengthening Your Marriage, Family, and Friendships by John Gottman. Three Rivers Press, 2002.

Difficult Conversations: How to Discuss What Matters Most by Douglas Stone, Bruce Patton, and Sheila Heen. Penguin Putnam, 1999.

Love is Never Enough: How Couples can Overcome Misunderstandings, Resolve Conflicts, and Solve Relationship

Problems through Cognitive Therapy by Aaron Beck, MD. Harper Collins, 1989.

Messages: The Communication Skills Book 2nd Ed by Matthew McKay, PhD, Martha Davis, PhD, and Patrick Fanning. New Harbinger Publications, 1995.

We Can Work It Out by Clifford Notarius, PhD and Howard Markman, PhD. Putnam, 1993.

Assertiveness Skills

When I Say No, I Feel Guilty by Manuel Smith, PhD, Bantam Books, 1975.

Your Perfect Right: Assertiveness and Equality in Your Life and Relationships (8th Ed.) by Robert Alberti, PhD and Michael Emmons, PhD. Impact Publishers, 2001.

Sexuality Issues

Becoming Orgasmic: A Sexual and Personal Growth Program for Women by Julie Heiman, PhD and Joseph LoPiccolo, PhD. Fireside, 1987.

For Each Other: Sharing Sexual Intimacy by Lonnie Barbach, PhD. Signet Books, 2001.

In Sickness and Health: Sex, Love, and Chronic Illness by Lucille Carlton. Delacorte Press, 1996.

The New Male Sexuality, Revised Edition by Bernie Zilbergeld, PhD. Bantam Books, 1999.

Notes

1   **Writing Out The Storm: Reading and Writing Your Way Through Serious Illness or Injury** by Barbara Abercrombie. St. Martin's Griffin, 2002. p. 131.

2   LIVESTRONG Poll Fact Sheet by the Lance Armstrong Foundation, November 30, 2004.

3   "Surviving Breast Cancer and Living with Lymphedema: Resiliency among Women in the Context of Their Families" by M. E. Radina and J. M. Armer. Journal of Family Nursing, 2004; 10:485-505.
    "Post Breast Cancer Lymphedema and the Family: A Qualitative Investigation of Families Coping with Chronic Illness" by M. E. Radina and J. M. Armer. Journal of Family Nursing, 2001; 7:281-299.

4   "Correlates of post traumatic growth in husbands of breast cancer survivors" by T. Weiss. Psychooncology. 2004; 13(4):260-68.

5   "Coping with the Disfiguring Effects of Vitiligo: A Preliminary Investigation into the Effects of Cognitive-behavioural Therapy" by L. Papadopoulos, R. Bor, and C. Legg. Br J Med Psychol 1999; 72:385-96.
    "A Preliminary Study of the Potential of Social Skills for Improving the Quality of Social Interaction for the Facially Disfigured" by N. Rumsey, R. Bull, and D. Gahagan. Soc Behav 1986; 1: 143-5.
    "An Evaluation of the Impact of Social Interaction Skills Training for Facially Disfigured People" by E. Robinson, N. Rumsey, and J. Partridge. Br J Plast Surg 1996; 49: 281-9.

6   "Lymphedema: Pathogenesis, Prevention, and Treatment" by P Marcks. Cancer Practice 1997, 5(1): 32-38. "Adjusting to Disfigurement: Processes Involved in Dealing with Being Visibly Different" by A Thompson and G Kent. Clinical Psychology Review, 2001, 21(5): 663-682.
    "Psychopathology and Psychological Problems in Patients with Burn Scars: Epidemiology and Management" by N Van Loey and M Van Son. American Journal of Clinical Dermatology, 2003, 4(4): 245-272.

Chapter 11:
Asking "Why?"

Normal Search for Meaning

Humans are thinking beings. It is our nature to look for patterns in events and to seek to understand our lives and our world. We struggle to make sense out of things that happen. We want to know "why?"—especially when something bad or unexpected occurs.

When you are first diagnosed, you try to make sense of that in order to come to terms with it. When symptoms fluctuate, you look for patterns. You need to come to grips with what it means to now have lymphedema for the rest of your life.

How do you fit this in with your view of yourself? You may wonder if you have failed or have done something wrong. You may feel defective. You may feel ashamed or feel guilty.

On a day-to-day, practical level, you try to figure out why your lymphedema improves or worsens. Taking effective action so you can exert control symptoms requires knowledge and understanding.

You seek answers to questions such as, *"What do these symptoms and physical changes mean? Which are signs of problems? What do I need to do? How do I know I'm on the right track—especially with a condition that can fluctuate unpredictably?"*

Sometimes, having lymphedema changes your view of other people. This can be a key issue if others are responsible for your condition and, particularly if you feel they were at fault in some way.

On the large scale, how does the fact of lymphedema fit with your religious beliefs, your philosophy of life, or your view of the world? How do you come to terms with an incurable condition? How do you accept uncertainty? How do you answer the question, "*Why me?*"

No one can tell you "the right answers" to these questions because each individual answers these questions differently.

I *can* tell you that the answers you come to, and the conclusions you draw, *will* guide your actions and will profoundly influence your emotions. Your search for meaning is important.

Common Questions

66 I used to ask 'why me?' Then one day I asked 'why not me?' and **99** it totally changed my attitude.

Many different questions may come to your mind. Check those that you have asked yourself:

☐ *"Why did this happen?"*

☐ *"What did I do to deserve lymphedema? Why me?"*

☐ *"Did I do something that contributed to this condition or to my complications?"*

☐ *"How does this affect my view of who I am as a person?"*

☐ *"Can I cope? Am I resilient or am I helpless?"*

☐ *"Did someone cause it? Could someone have prevented it? Whose fault is it?"*

☐ *"How is this affecting my view of other people?"*

☐ *"How does this affect my view of my future?"*

☐ *"How can this fit my sense of justice and fairness?"*

☐ *"Why am I ill when others are healthy?"*

☐ *"How does having lymphedema fit my religious or philosophical beliefs?"*

☐ *"How does having lymphedema fit with a belief in a just and loving God?"*

☐ *"Is God punishing me?"*

☐ *"Has this changed my view of the world?"*

If other questions of a similar nature have troubled you, write those down. In particular, write down any questions that still bother you.

_____

_____

Raising questions is a healthy human reaction. It is a universal human urge to seek answers. We seek answers that help us to come to terms with what has happened.

How can we acknowledge the negative and move forward constructively? Many books have been written about this issue. One of the most popular books to address this topic is **When Bad Things Happen to Good People** (see **Resources**).

Benefits of the Search for Meaning

Grappling with such questions can be painful. It helps to realize that, over time, rewards can come as a result. These rewards include:

- ☐ Learning what worsens or improves your lymphedema
- ☐ Identifying problems and their solutions
- ☐ Making necessary, healthy changes, physically and/or emotionally
- ☐ Increasing in assertiveness, self-respect, and self-reliance
- ☐ Growing in maturity and wisdom
- ☐ Gaining increased empathy, tolerance, forgiveness, and acceptance
- ☐ Deepening or renewing your religious faith or set of guiding beliefs

Check the boxes above if you have already begun to notice any of these changes.

Write down other rewards that you have gained, or hope to gain, through your search to make meaning out of your experience of lymphedema on the lines below.

_____

_____

Pause and reflect. What have you done that has made these gains possible? What steps can you take next?

_____

_____

Problematic Responses to the Search for Meaning

It is the difficult times that stretch us, not the easy times. Grappling with hard questions such as those above and seeking answers to them is a normal, healthy, predictable response.

At times, the healthy search for meaning can get derailed. You may have trouble finding answers or you may reach conclusions that sustain emotional distress and make it hard for you to come to peace with the changed reality.

Signs that the normal search for meaning has become derailed can include:

- Loss of meaning or faith
- Focus on self-blame, guilt, or shame
- Focus on blaming others

Loss of Meaning or Faith

A loss of meaning or faith occurs when you can't fit the reality of lymphedema into the life view or religious belief that helps you make sense of things. Your faith in God, or in God's goodness, may falter. Your faith and trust in a higher power may feel lost. Your belief in the principles that have guided your life and given it meaning may be shaken.

You can come to believe that your philosophy of life, or your religious belief, is invalid. You may feel you have nothing to replace them. Here are some signals that this may be happening. Check any boxes that apply to you.

☐ You find yourself unable to come to terms with what has happened to you. It seems wrong or unfair in some fundamental way that you cannot accept.

☐ You have lost your belief that the world makes sense. You feel that life is meaningless.

☐ This has shaken your previous religious belief in the existence of God (or a higher power).

☐ If you have (or had) a religious faith, you now believe that God is punishing you. Or you now believe that God is unjust, malevolent, or uncaring.

Write down any other problematic conclusions that reflect a loss of meaning or faith.

Write down any ideas that come to you right now about what you can do to address these losses. If you have no ideas now, let yourself think about this in the back of your mind as you read the rest of this chapter. This may be the beginning of a journey of exploration which leads to deeper wisdom and understanding.

Part of the Human Condition

We all experience pain, sorrow, and struggle at some time. This is an inescapable fact of life. As the old saying goes, *"Into each life, some rain must fall."*

- **Occasional showers.** Some lucky people have only rare, brief, showers and they are able to recover quickly.

- **Scattered storms.** Many of us have heavy showers but with enough time between them for recovery.

- **Stormy Weather.** And some of us just have the unfortunate luck to have times where heavy storms seem to come one after another, dumping buckets of rain right on our heads, until we feel as if we are drowning.[1]

If you fall into that last category, examine your coping techniques, your living situation, and your lymphedema care. Are your thoughts, actions, or inaction putting you at risk for health, psychological, interpersonal, or other problems?

If current thoughts or actions put you at risk, weigh the costs. If you continue on your current course of action or inaction, what results do you expect? What are the best and the worst outcomes to be expected if you follow the same course? If you change? What can you improve?

Past experiences and actions do not have to predict the present and future. You can go through times when it seems as though only bad happens to you. Yet you can survive to overcome and thrive.

Rebuilding

Life is not always fair or just. Terrible things can happen to wonderful people who have done nothing to "deserve" them. This can shake your fundamental beliefs.

Despite this unfairness, your challenge is still the same: to create a meaningful life for yourself with satisfactions, despite whatever may have happened. You search for a source of hope, faith, and meaning.

Everyone struggles with these issues at times. You have lots of company on this journey. Each of us must find his or her personal belief. The answer or conclusion that satisfies one person may not satisfy another. You must find the answer that is right for you.

Coping Suggestions:

Remind yourself that people have overcome all kinds of tragedies. Learn from them. You may want to read autobiographies, paying attention to how the author found meaning or faith.

Review the ideas in this chapter. If you cannot resolve these troubling questions or you keep going in circles, talk to someone you trust.

The person to whom you turn should be someone who supports your spiritual, religious, or philosophical beliefs—even if they don't share them.

You may turn to a wise friend, a religious adviser, a spiritual counselor, or a psychotherapist who is knowledgeable about the search for meaning.

Focus on Blame

We have just discussed one problematic conclusion to the search for meaning: loss of faith. Another harmful response is to focus your energies on placing blame rather than on coming to terms with the reality and moving forward. You can become mired in blaming yourself or others.

Self-Blame

The following are examples of blaming yourself. Check any boxes that apply to you.

☐ "I did something wrong. I made bad decisions or was in the wrong place at the wrong time. It's my fault that I have lymphedema, and so I deserve to suffer."

☐ "I must have some need to be ill. I'm causing this somehow."

☐ "My child has primary lymphedema. I caused this and I'll never forgive myself."

☐ "It's wrong to feel sorry for myself because I should never have negative emotions."

☐ "I can't cope. I can't change. I'm just useless and weak."

Write down any other problematic conclusions or thoughts that reflect self-blame.

_____

_____

How does self-blame make you feel? Do you like the results? Has it led to positive changes?

_____

_____

Problems With Self-Blame

You may simply assume that whenever something bad happens it must be your fault. This is called *"blaming the victim."*

Automatic self-blame interferes with thinking clearly. It makes you feel bad. It is not helpful. Objectively evaluate the facts. Look for other contributing factors.

Blaming yourself for your natural emotional reactions doesn't make sense either. It just makes you feel worse. Your job is to face the challenge and overcome it, not to blame yourself for having it.

Of course, sometimes people do contribute to their own emotional distress or physical problems. Children may inherit lymphedema from their parents. What if you have grounds for self-blame? What if you did do, or continue to do, things that cause or worsen lymphedema?

What If I Really Am To Blame?

Look back at the results of self-blaming in your answers to the questions above. Do you like what you see? Is self-blame, however justified, creating positive results?

Consider the following:

- Blame doesn't change the past. The past is past. It is not open to change.

- You were not perfect in the past. Achieving or maintain perfection is not possible. Your first challenge is to accept this fact.

- Now consider another key fact: Improvement is possible. The future is open to change. You are influencing it now. It is affected by your choices in the present, day by day, choice by choice.

- Your second challenge is to learn and act on the lessons from the past that will help you create a better future for yourself.

Past mistakes and present imperfections do not take away your responsibility to care for yourself the best way you can. You don't have to be perfect to make things better. With each daily decision, you have a fresh chance to make choices and move on.

Blaming Others

Here are some warning signals that your search for meaning has been hijacked into blame directed toward others. Check the items that you find yourself thinking about repeatedly:

☐ The actions of others and how they caused or worsened your lymphedema.

☐ The limitations, flaws, shortcoming, and mistakes of other people.

☐ The ways in which other people let you down.

Write down any other conclusions or thoughts that focus on blaming others.

_____

_____

How does blame make you feel? Do you like the results? Has it led to positive changes?

_____

_____

Problems with Blaming Others

When your search for meaning gets derailed, it harms you. Whether you blame yourself or others, simply focusing on blame changes nothing *and* it can leave you bitter and disheartened.

Just as you are not perfect, other people are not perfect. People can be thoughtless, selfish, and uncaring. They may be ignorant, misinformed, or irresponsible. They can make bad choices, poor decisions, and tragic mistakes.

Most of the time, most people are trying to do their best, just as you are trying to do your best. Like you, they are hampered by their limitations, their past, their personalities, and the limits of their knowledge.

You do not know what other people struggle with inside. You do not know what is behind the façade of their public lives.

What If Others Really Are To Blame?

Sometimes others *are* at fault. When this is the case, look at all the facts and the big picture:

- If you have primary lymphedema, you may *have* inherited it from your parents – along with many other attributes, good and bad. It is impossible to predict in advance the exact combination of genes that any one child will inherit.

- If you developed secondary lymphedema as a result of medical care for cancer or some other condition, the treatment that caused your lymphedema may also have saved your life. Was the treatment or diagnostic procedure that resulted in lymphedema undertaken because it was believed, at the time, to be appropriate care?

- If you developed secondary lymphedema as a consequence of some other medical condition (such as paralysis, obesity, circulatory problems, etc.) is there really anyone to blame? Could anything have been done differently with the information available at the time?

- If you have secondary lymphedema as a result of an accident or injury, was someone at fault? Could the accident have been prevented?

Look at your options. Consider talking to people who are experts in this area and whom you trust to be both knowledgeable and objective. Ask them questions such as, *"Can I have the mistakes corrected or be compensated?" "If I try to get compensation, how likely am I to be successful?" "What will it cost me in terms of money, time, energy, resources, and mental anguish?" "What is the most likely end result and is it worth the cost?"*

Think long and hard about the facts that:

- Others are imperfect.

- Mistakes and tragedies occur.

- Life was never guaranteed to be fair.

Where Does This Leave You?

Review what you have written so far in this chapter. What have you learned about the emotional effects of blaming?

Separate action from blame. Think about how you can correct problems while causing yourself the least emotional distress.

Coping Suggestions:

Regardless of who was at fault, minimize the energy you spend blaming - yourself or others. After all, the past is gone. Blame doesn't change the past.

Save your energy for constructive action.

Focus on what is possible.

Let the facts guide your actions.

Your Conclusions and Their Impact on Your Life

Think about your answers to the questions in this chapter. Use what you have learned to complete Worksheet 11-1: Searching for Meaning:

- In the left hand column, write the questions that have been, or continue to be, important in your search for meaning.

- In the middle column, write your answers or conclusions regarding each question.

- In the right hand column, write about the impact of each conclusion on your life, negative or positive.

For the questions you have answered, how satisfied are you with your conclusions?

_____

_____

If you are struggling with important unanswered questions or problematic conclusions, what impact does this have on your ability to cope with lymphedema and thrive emotionally?

_____

_____

Now, turn to Worksheet 14-2: **My Emotional Challenges** on page 201 and complete the line for "Searching for meaning."

Worksheet 11-1: Searching for Meaning

Questions	My Answers Or Conclusions	Impact On My Life

Resources

When Bad Things Happen to Good People by Harold Kushner. Avon Books, 1981.

Notes

1   Adapted from **Overcoming Post-Traumatic Stress Disorder—Client Manual** by Larry Smyth, PhD. New Harbinger Publications, 1999.

Chapter 12

Lessons from Your Past

You may think of the past as being over and done with—but past events, and the lessons learned in the past, can help or hinder you as you cope with lymphedema.

The first half of this chapter discusses trauma and common responses to traumatic events. The second half of the chapter discusses how our "core beliefs," general beliefs about life stemming from our past, can be helpful or unhelpful.

Trauma

Many people develop lymphedema as a result of life-threatening illness or a serious accident. Even if trauma did not cause your lymphedema, other difficult or traumatic events experienced in the course of your life may affect your response to lymphedema now.

Some of the information that immediately follows may not apply to you. Read whatever does apply and feel free to skip the rest.

No matter what caused your lymphedema, be sure to read the section on General Lessons from the Past: Core Beliefs. This section applies to everyone.

Lymphedema-Related Traumatic Events

If your lymphedema was caused by cancer treatment, a life-threatening illness, a serious accident, or some other traumatic event, work through this section.

Write down the events that resulted in your lymphedema:

_____

Other Traumatic Events

Have you had other past experiences that were difficult or traumatic? These may include:

☐ Being verbally or physically threatened

☐ Being verbally or physically abused or assaulted

☐ Being sexually abused, molested, or raped

☐ Witnessing violence

☐ Fearing for your life and safety or for someone else's life and safety

☐ The death or serious illness of a loved one, especially if you witnessed it

☐ Growing up in difficult circumstances, such as with a substance-abusing parent, in a dangerous neighborhood, in unstable family situation, etc.

Check off all that apply to you. If you have had other particularly difficult or traumatic experiences, list them here:

_____

Past events can affect your reactions to present challenges. You are more likely to have more severe or long-lasting responses to lymphedema-related trauma if you have experienced other past traumas.

At the same time, difficult or painful past experiences are not purely negative. They can result in strong coping skills, resilience, confidence, pride, maturity, empathy, determination, wisdom and many other positives.[1]

The Impact of Traumas

Every single one of us is likely to notice effects when we have, or witness, traumatic experiences. It has nothing to do with being weak or strong.

Traumas tend to have more negative impact if the experience was severe and/or long lasting and you have experienced other significant traumatic events. You are also more likely to have more trouble overcoming traumas if

Sam's Story

It is amazing how smells can bring back memories. Once while we were touring a safety lab I smelled smoke and suddenly I was back in the fire where I got hurt. Not just reminded of the fire, I was back there in that fire. I could see the flames and feel the heat. I dropped into a crouch and started yelling 'it's going to fall' and pushing everyone out, just like I did before I got hurt.

Fortunately one of the guys with me had been in the war and knew about flashbacks. He kept talking to me calmly, led me outside, and made me look at the sky and the sunshine. I was shaking and it took me a long time to calm down and realize what happened. Then I got really scared that I was losing my mind. I've dreamed about that fire a million times but this was so real and so sudden that it frightened me.

My friend told me not to worry and that he had been through this after the war. The first flashback is the scariest and having flash-backs does not mean that you are crazy. He'd found that seeing a therapist at the VA really helped. He said that if you get help, the flashbacks happen less and you can control them better. He also told me that getting help is really important, some of his Army buddies didn't and they are still having a tough time.

your support network is weak, if you only have a few coping skills, or if you have a generally negative outlook on life.

Check the items that pertain to you:

☐ The trauma and/or its consequences were severe.

☐ The trauma and/or its consequences lasted a long time.

☐ Your support network is limited, unavailable, or of poor quality.

☐ Your coping skills are limited, unhelpful, or overwhelmed.

☐ Your personality tends to be negative, pessimistic, or angry.

☐ Your emotional state overall is characterized by distress or negative emotions.

☐ You have experienced other traumas.

Normal Response to Traumas

Remember how you felt when you were diagnosed with lymphedema? Remember what it was like dealing with the cause of your lymphedema? Remember any other traumatic experiences you have survived?

Recall how you felt and what you did during those times. How many of these normal responses to trauma have you experienced? Did you:

- ☐ Feel the need to think about it and talk about it over and over?

- ☐ Find yourself reliving certain aspects in great detail or being unable to recall other details?

- ☐ Notice that you were jumpy, teary, or irritable during the day or had nightmares or insomnia at night?

- ☐ Alternate between needing to think or talk about what happened and wanting to avoid it entirely?

- ☐ Experience being flooded with emotions at some times and feeling emotionally numb at other times?

Traumatic experiences can trigger some or all of the above reactions. This is especially true for traumatic experiences that carry the potential for death or serious injury and that result in intense fear, helplessness, or horror. Facing the possibility of death is traumatic for **anyone**.

Take a second to really think about this. You and I don't generally confront the fact of our mortality head on. Intellectually, we all know that we will eventually die, but we don't usually think about it. Most of the time, we go through our daily tasks from day to day assuming that we will be alive tomorrow or next week.

Trauma challenges this assumption. Traumatic events can also shake the assumption that most people are basically well meaning. They can upset the belief that your immediate world is safe.

Traumatic events can powerfully affect memory and emotions. Different people react to trauma differently. When emotional healing proceeds normally, the intensity of your emotional reaction (or numbness) lessens over time.

You find yourself more able to choose when and what you remember. The shock and horror recede into the background. You move forward with life.

To quote from research on women with lymphedema after breast cancer: *"Despite the fact that managing both chronic lymphedema and breast cancer survival was distressing ..., most women were able to carry on with their lives."*[2]

For some people, the trauma fades into the background relatively quickly and easily. For others, healing takes more time and more work.

Your goal is to work through the emotional reactions. You want to regain a sense of yourself as competent and coping, not helpless and threatened. You want the perspective that the world contains tragedy and challenge, but also joy and mastery. Here are some specific suggestions:

Coping Suggestions:

Restart daily life. Do things that give you pleasure or a sense of accomplishment.

Connect with other people and with your community. Don't isolate yourself.

Get the information or practical help you need to feel more in control and able to cope.

Schedule times that you can spend writing about past events that trouble you. Repeatedly review the event in a deliberate, prolonged, thoughtful manner. Focus on the positives that have (or could) come from the event.

If you notice you're avoiding something because of the traumatic experience, deliberately stop avoiding and confront it until it bothers you less.

Use the skills you will learn in Chapters 16 and 17.

Problematic Response to Traumas

Your natural response becomes problematic when you can't move forward. You can't seem to emotionally process the trauma and become stuck in a loop of distress.

The traumatic memories or emotions replay endlessly. You can't relax, you can't experience the full range of joyful emotions, and you shut down or avoid anything that triggers trauma-related memories.

Do you have any of these signs?

☐ Do you find yourself remembering or reliving the trauma, over and over, with continuing distress?

☐ Do you continue for weeks to have physical symptoms of over-reactivity, such as insomnia, an exaggerated startle response, trouble relaxing or concentrating, or reacting irritably?

☐ Do you feel as though you are cut off from your normal range of emotions?

☐ Do you feel emotionally detached from other people?

☐ Do you have an ongoing lack of interest in things that would normally interest you?

☐ Do you persistently avoid anything that reminds you of the trauma because you are fearful of the intense emotions you would feel?

If you checked one or more of the boxes, use the coping suggestions above.

If you have checked most or all of the boxes and these signs only began after a traumatic experience, you may be having an understandable response called *post-traumatic stress disorder (PTSD)*. If using the coping suggestions above does not result in change, consult a licensed mental health professional trained and experienced in treating PTSD.

You do not have to remain trapped. There are specific psychotherapy treatments and medications that can help. Seek them out.

The Good News about Traumatic Past Events

Because so much psychological research focuses on problems, you can get the impression that your past controls your present and future. This is simply not true.

Human beings have extraordinary capacities for resilience. Our past is not our destiny. Research on particularly vulnerable children in very difficult situations found that "...*resilience is common* ...".[3]

No matter what past traumas you may have experienced, things can improve. You can learn to cope more effectively. Trauma-related emotional reactions can occur less often and be less intense. You can grow in confidence and ability to manage whatever reactions remain.

Positive changes can result. You can achieve increased spirituality, deeper awareness of your core values, closer connections to others, commitment to positive life changes, and increased wisdom, integrity, and honesty.

Your past *can* influence you. However, it does *not* control you or determine what you do in the future. What happened in the past is far less important than what you do in the present.

At the end of this chapter (on page 170) , you will find Worksheet 12-7: The Impact of Traumatic Events. List the traumas you have experienced and survived. Think about the negative and the positive consequences or aspects of your experience and write those down.

General Lessons from the Past: Core Beliefs

Chapter 11: Searching for Meaning discussed the fact that we all, as human beings, try to make sense out of everything that happens to us. We actively draw lessons or beliefs about life from our experiences and from other people. We draw conclusions about what to expect and how to react to problems.

Each of us has basic beliefs or expectations about ourselves, about other people, and about the world. These are beliefs that seem obviously true to us, that we believe deep inside, in our gut, in our core. Such general beliefs are known as "*core beliefs.*" Different people have different core beliefs.

Our core beliefs are shaped by our past experiences. They are general lessons learned from the past. So, in this way, our past affects our present because of its effect of these beliefs.

Core beliefs act as a kind of automatic filter. They affect what we notice and remember. They affect how we interpret and react to events. They are like standing instructions about what to ignore and what to file as important and relevant.

We notice those things that *fit* our beliefs. We tend to ignore or forget those things that *don't* fit our beliefs.

We interpret what happens in ways that match our beliefs. Unless we become aware of it and change it, this automatic filtering occurs without our awareness.

For example if I believe deep down inside that I am a hopeless failure, I will discount any success as a fluke. I will perceive every minor flaw or failure as proof that I am incompetent—just as I expected. Positive and negative experiences are made to fit my core belief about myself.

If, on the other hand, I believe deep inside that I am a resilient survivor who copes, then I see every success as evidence of my abilities. I interpret each failure as a temporary stepping stone to eventual success; or I see it as caused by factors other than me. Again, positive and negative experiences are viewed in ways that fit my core belief.

Helpful Core Beliefs

As you saw in the example above, core beliefs can be helpful or unhelpful. Your core beliefs affect how you act, and react, when faced with challenges.

For example, if you believe you can succeed, that others may help, and that problems can be resolved, you will work hard, look for other people to help, and remain optimistic. Many famous sayings reflect underlying helpful core beliefs, for example:

- *"When the going gets tough, the tough get going."*
- *"It's always darkest before the dawn."*
- *"All things are possible for those who love the Lord."*
- *"When one door closes, another opens."*
- *"When you get to the end of your rope, tie a knot and hold on."*

The next three worksheets give examples of helpful core beliefs. There are three worksheets so you can rate beliefs about three areas:

1. Yourself
2. Other people
3. The world and life in general

Rate how much you personally feel each belief is true. Base your ratings on your gut reaction, not your intellectual thought.

Helpful Core Beliefs about Myself Worksheet

Worksheet 12-1 presents core beliefs for how you think about yourself.

For each core belief statement in the first column, rate the degree to which you believe the statement is true. Use a scale of 0 – 10 where 0 is not at all true or believable and 10 is completely true. Base your rating on your "gut reaction." Write whatever number comes to your mind.

If there are other helpful core beliefs about yourself that you believe, or would like to believe, write them in the bottom part of the worksheet and rate them as well.

Helpful Core Beliefs about Others Worksheet

Worksheet 12-2 presents core beliefs about other people.

For each core belief in the first column, write a number from 0 – 10 in the second column rating how much you believe, in your heart, that the statement is true. Base your rating on your "gut reaction". Write whatever number comes to your mind.

If there are other helpful core beliefs about other people that you believe, or would like to believe, write them in at the bottom and rate them as well.

Helpful Core Beliefs about the World Worksheet

Worksheet 12-3 presents core beliefs about the world and life in general.

For each core belief in the first column, write a number from 0 – 10 in the second column rating how much you believe, in your heart, that the statement is true. Base your rating on your gut reaction. Write whatever number comes to your mind.

If there are other helpful core beliefs about the world and life in general that you believe, or would like to believe, write them in at the bottom and rate them as well.

Notice your helpful core beliefs, especially the ones you currently rated 7 or higher in the worksheets. Think about their impact on your life, your emotions, and your response to lymphedema. You can write this down in Worksheet 12-8: The Impact of Core Beliefs on page 171.

Drawing on Positive Core Beliefs

If you rated generally 7 or higher on most of the helpful core beliefs, congratulations! Your core beliefs will help you as you face the challenges posed by lymphedema. The more positive your core beliefs, the more optimistic, confident, and satisfied you will feel. Helpful core beliefs are a tremendous asset in surmounting the difficulties of life with lymphedema.

Coping Suggestions:

Notice every event in your life, no matter how small, that supports the positive beliefs.

Reflect on these beliefs.

Act according to them when you deal with the effects of lymphedema.

Draw strength from them.

Strengthening Positive Core Beliefs

If you rated 6 or lower on several of the helpful core beliefs, reflect for a moment about what may be causing your relatively low ratings. If you think your ratings reflect a temporary problem or mood, redo them in a day or two.

Sometimes ratings reflect a current life problem. Actively work to resolve or leave situations that undermine helpful beliefs. If other people are mistreating you or if your living situation is dangerous, address these real-life problems. *Then* work on your core beliefs.

On the other hand, if it is your *perception* of reality—not reality itself—that is the problem, change your core beliefs using these suggestions. This can take time but can pay big dividends.

Worksheet 12-1: Helpful Core Beliefs about Myself

Core Belief	Degree I Believe It
I am lovable.	
I am able to cope.	
I am competent and capable.	
I have a right to happiness.	
I can enjoy things.	
I can persevere even when something is difficult.	
I am a caring person.	
I am smart.	
I deserve respect.	
I am a good human being.	
I am resilient.	
I can overcome challenges.	

Worksheet 12-2: Helpful Core Beliefs about Others

Core Belief	Degree I Believe It
Other people are generally well meaning.	
Most people in my life can be trusted.	
Most people in my life are caring.	
Other people are doing the best they can.	
Others can be a source of help.	
Others can be a source of support.	

Worksheet 12-3: Helpful Core Beliefs about the World and Life in General

Core Belief	Degree I Believe It
My world is generally safe.	
Things usually work out.	
Problems can be resolved, overcome, or coped with.	
Despite its problems, life has meaning.	
Despite its problems, life has pleasures.	

Coping Suggestions:

Select helpful core belief(s) you want to strengthen. Start a journal or notebook in which you write about this belief.

Start by writing down in your journal or notebook every past experience that supports this positive core belief. Add more as you remember them.

In your daily life, actively look for evidence that supports the new belief.

At the end of the day, write those experiences, no matter how small, that provide more evidence that this core belief is true or helpful.

At the beginning or end of the day, reread what you have written so far.

Mark your calendar to recheck once a month and measure whether your conviction that this helpful core belief is true has increased. Re-rate the belief using the worksheet. You should see progress over several months.

Problematic Core Beliefs

Core beliefs may come from our past experiences but, once established, they automatically affect our present reactions – rather like software programs installed on a computer. You want to strengthen your helpful beliefs and weaken your problematic beliefs. To change problematic beliefs, you have to identify them.

Problematic Core Beliefs about Yourself Worksheet

Worksheet 12-4 presents core beliefs about yourself.

For each core belief in the first column, write a number in the second column that rates on a scale of 0-10 how much you believe, in your heart, that the statement is true. Base your rating on your "gut reaction". Write whatever number comes to your mind.

If you have other negative, problematic core beliefs about yourself, write them in at the bottom and rate them as well.

Problematic Core Beliefs about Others Worksheet

Worksheet 12-5 presents core beliefs about other people.

For each core belief in the first column, write a number from 0 – 10 in the second column rating how much you believe, in your heart, that the statement is true. Base your rating on your "gut reaction". Write whatever number comes to your mind.

If you have other problematic core beliefs about other people, write them in at the bottom of the worksheet and rate them as well.

Problematic Core Beliefs about the World Worksheet

Worksheet 12-6 presents core beliefs about the world and life in general.

For each core belief in the first column, write a number from 0 – 10 in the second column rating how much you believe, in your heart, that the statement is true. Base your rating on your "gut reaction". Write whatever number comes to your mind.

If you have other problematic core beliefs about the world or life in general, write them in at the bottom and rate them as well.

The higher your ratings, the more these beliefs will lower your mood, interfere with the quality of your life, and disrupt your attempts to overcome lymphedema's challenges.

Review any strongly held problematic core beliefs. Think about their impact on your life, your emotions, and your response to lymphedema. Think about your reasons to challenge and change these beliefs. Write this down in Worksheet 12-8: The Impact of Core Beliefs on page 171.

Changing Unhelpful Beliefs

Unhelpful core beliefs *can* be modified. Their impact on your life can lessen.

Two self-help workbooks have particularly good information about changing core beliefs. One is **Mind Over Mood** by Drs. Greenberger and Padesky. The other is **Reinventing Your Life** by Drs. Young and Klosko.

Worksheet 12-4: Problematic Core Beliefs about Myself

Core Belief	Degree I Believe It
I am unlovable.	
I am fragile and helpless.	
I am incompetent. I'm a screw-up.	
I am worthless.	
I will never have happiness.	
I always give up. I can't do anything hard. I am weak.	
I am a hopeless failure.	
I don't deserve anything.	
I am stupid.	
I don't deserve respect.	
I am a bad person.	
I can't cope.	
I can't deal with challenges.	

Worksheet 12-5: Problematic Core Beliefs about Others

Core Belief	Degree I Believe It
Other people are only out for all they can get. They are selfish, and are only interested in their own agenda.	
People in my life can't be trusted.	
People in my life don't care.	
People do the least they can get away with.	
Others are useless and unhelpful.	
Others are unsupportive and don't understand.	

Worksheet 12-6: Problematic Core Beliefs about the World

Core Belief	Degree I Believe It
The whole world is threatening and dangerous. Don't ever let your guard down because something will always go wrong.	
Bad things always happen. Good things never last.	
Problems are overwhelming and unsolvable. It's hopeless.	
What's the point? What I do doesn't matter. I can't make a difference.	
Life is toil and trouble. Any pleasures are outweighed by the problems.	

You may also find this book helpful: **Successful Problem-Solving: A Workbook to Overcome the Four Core Beliefs That Keep You Stuck** by Matthew McKay, PhD. and Patrick Fanning.

It has been estimated that this kind of change can take 6 months of active effort or longer.[4] You may find it helpful to work with a licensed psychotherapist who is experienced and trained in this type of therapy. Psychotherapy groups, self-help support groups, and other sources of support for change can also help.

The Past and Its Impact on Your Life

Review your answers to the questions, checklists, and worksheets in this chapter.

If you haven't already done so, write what you have learned in the worksheets below. Worksheet 12-7 deals with the impact of traumas. Worksheet 12-8 deals with the impact of core beliefs.

The Impact of Traumatic Events Worksheet

List traumatic events you have experienced in the left column,

Next, write the negatives have resulted from these events in the center column.

Now, deliberately take a broader focus. Move away from thinking about losses and negatives. Think about what still remains in your life. Look for gains that have occurred in your life despite the losses (or even as a result of them). What positives have resulted? Write those in the right column.

The Impact of Core Beliefs Worksheet

Review your helpful and problematic core beliefs in the worksheets above. What impact do these core beliefs have on you and on your ability to deal with lymphedema? How do they affect your response to the emotional challenges of lymphedema? Write your answers in the worksheet.

Now, turn to Worksheet 14-2: **My Emotional Challenges** on page 201 and complete the line for "Trauma and Core Beliefs."

Worksheet 12-7: The Impact of Traumatic Events

Traumatic Events	Negatives That Resulted	Positives That Remain or That Resulted

Worksheet 12-8: The Impact of Core Beliefs

Impact Of Problematic Core Beliefs											
Impact Of Helpful Core Beliefs											

Resources

Core Beliefs Resources

Reinventing Your Life: The Breakthrough Program to End Negative Behavior…And Feel Great Again by Jeffrey Young, PhD and Janet Klosko, PhD. Plume Books, 1994.

Mind Over Mood: Change How You Feel by Changing the Way You Think by Dennis Greenberger, PhD and Christine Padesky, PhD. Guilford Publications, 1995.

Successful Problem-Solving: A Workbook To Overcome The Four Core Beliefs That Keep You Stuck by Matthew McKay, PhD and Patrick Fanning. New Harbinger Publications, 2002.

Trauma and PTSD Resources

Opening Up: The Healing Power Of Expressing Emotions by James Pennebaker, PhD. The Guilford Press, 1997.

Overcoming Post-Traumatic Stress Disorder—Client Manual by Larry Smyth, PhD. New Harbinger Publications, 1999.

Writing To Heal: A Guided Journal For Recovering From Trauma And Emotional Upheaval by James Pennebaker, PhD. New Harbinger Publications, 2004.

Notes

1   Kornblith AB, Ligibel J: Psychosocial and sexual functioning of survivors of breast cancer. Semin Oncol 30(6): 799-813, 2003.

2   "Women's Experience of Lymphedema" by Carter, B. J. *Oncology Nursing Forum* 1997; 24: 880.

3   "Loss, Trauma, and Human Resilience: Have We Underestimated the Human Capacity to Thrive after Extremely Aversive Events?" by Bonanno, G. *American Psychologist.* January 2004; vol. 59 no. 1: 20-28.

4   **Mind Over Mood: Change How You Feel by Changing the Way You Think** by Dennis Greenberger, PhD and Christine Padesky, PhD. Guilford Publications, 1995.

Chapter 13

Current Life Stresses

Lymphedema occurs in the context of the rest of your life. It brings its own stresses. Your daily life may also present sources of stress.

The good news is that just the fact that you have stress in your life is not the whole story. Your resources and your skill in dealing with stress are equally, if not more, important.

Therefore, this chapter starts by having you identify positives in your life. You can use these positives to cope with or resolve stressors. They can help you take care of yourself and buffer you against the potential negative impact of stress.

The chapter goes on to review both predictably common and less common, more severe stresses. As you identify your stresses, you can use Worksheet 13-2: Taking Care of Myself (on page 187) to evaluate your current coping and, if you wish, plan ways to improve.

Positives in the Present

Let's start with the positives: your strengths, your supports, your skills, and your resources. In Chapter 12, you identified your core beliefs that are helpful. Now look at other helpful factors that are present in your life.

Deliberately noticing positives in your life improves your mood and fosters positive feelings such as gratitude and appreciation. Concentrating on the positive helps you thrive physically and emotionally despite lymphedema.

Lymphedema-Related Positives

Positives can be specifically lymphedema-related. What positives have entered your life as a result of lymphedema? These could include:

- Finding people who are knowledgeable about lymphedema.

- Locating reliable sources of information about lymphedema.

- Gaining lymphedema knowledge and self-care skills.

- Having effective lymphedema care products

- Meeting healthcare professionals and others who are supportive, caring, helpful or inspiring.

- Seeing the results of effective treatment.

- Making changes in lifestyle or activities that improve your general health. These may include regular exercise, controlling your weight, making healthy eating choices, and giving up poor health habits such as smoking.

Add any others that come to mind.
Note them all on Worksheet 13-1: Positives in the Present.

Other Positives

Now identify other positives. These can be positives about you personally, about people around you, or anything about your life and situation. Here are some examples:

- General personal traits, such as optimism, confidence, belief in yourself, energy, intelligence, creativity, problem-solving ability, determination, the ability to learn, helpful core beliefs, faith, gratitude, perseverance, etc.

- Sources of joy or pleasure.

- Activities that absorb and engross you.

- Accomplishments, achievement, or other sources of pride and self-worth.

- Relaxing activities or other things that reduce stress or help you cope.

- Caring family.

- Friends, neighbors, coworkers, and other people whom you value or appreciate.

- A safe living situation.

- Sources of income, insurance, practical assistance, etc.

- Community resources.

Add any others that come to mind.
Note them all on Worksheet 13-1: Positives in the Present.

Positives in the Present Worksheet

Make a comprehensive list of as many positive factors as you can think of, whether internal or external, emotional or practical, large or small using the worksheet on page 177. Add others as you think of them.

Coping Suggestions:

Review your list of positive factors daily, weekly, or monthly.

When you notice a new positive in your life, add it to your list.

Find ways to use these positives to reach your physical or emotional goals.

For example, maybe you have people to talk to when you feel angry, sad, scared, uncertain, or overwhelmed. Maybe you have activities that lift your mood, make you feel proud and self-confidence, and give you reasons to care for your emotional and physical health. Your literacy, intelligence, and self-awareness make change possible.

Positives can help you overcome the stresses in your life, whether mild or severe, whether lymphedema-related or not.

Normal Daily Life Stresses

Other life challenges don't stop just because you have lymphedema. Unfair though it seems, you don't get a pass on other life demands when you have a chronic condition. You still face normal life stresses.

You may be dealing with the stresses of work or school. You may be juggling many demands on your time.

> **❝** I don't think I am taking very good care of myself because I push so hard. I feel like everyone needs me to take care of them. Between the kids and the job and the house and the lymphedema, who takes care of me? The only way I get some down time is when I get sick. **❞**

You may have relationship or family stresses. You may be caring for children, parents, and/or a spouse. You may be coping with interpersonal stresses such as dating or dealing with coworkers, friends, or neighbors.

Turn to Worksheet 13-2: Taking Care Of Myself, on page 187. In the first column, list normal stresses in your life that you have identified.

How do you successfully cope with normal everyday stresses? You may use relaxation techniques, stress-management, and/or time management. You may prioritize, delegate, organize, and/or simplify. You may get emotional or physical help. You may build healthy activities into your schedule such as exercise, good nutrition, sleep, pleasure, etc.

List how you currently handle these stresses in the second column of Worksheet 13-2.

Using the 0-10 scale, mark how satisfied you are with your current coping in the third column.

Are there any other strengths, resources, positives, and skills that you could use? Write down changes that will improve your life or your emotions in the fourth column.

Common Lymphedema-Related Stresses

Now let's turn to lymphedema-related stresses. These vary from person-to-person. The list below includes a range of stresses from normal, predictable stresses to more severe, problematic stresses. Check off those that are present in your life:

☐ You have to learn about lymphedema and new ways of doing things.

☐ You spend time finding and going to lymphedema treatment.

☐ You have to make time to do your self-care routine.

Worksheet 13-1: Positives in the Present

Positives in the Present

☐ You have to wear hot and bulky bandages or compression garments.

☐ Sometimes you can't wear your wedding ring or your usual jewelry, clothing, or shoes.

☐ You have to cope with insurance to get reimbursement for treatment.

☐ You have to adapt your activities because of lymphedema.

☐ Sleep is disrupted because of bandaging or compression garments.

☐ You have no one at home who is able, or willing, to help you.

☐ Some days you seem to have little or no energy.

☐ You lose income because of lost work time or lymphedema-related disability.

☐ You are in debt for lymphedema-related expenses that are not covered by your insurance.

☐ You feel trapped in your current job by fear of losing your insurance coverage if you change jobs.

☐ You lost a job or promotion for a lymphedema-related reason.

☐ You are in chronic pain and poor health due to frequent infections and other lymphedema-related complications.

☐ You have less mobility due to swelling or lymphedema-related joint damage.

☐ You are on disability due to health reasons.

Add the stresses you checked, and any others that come to mind, in the first column of Worksheet 13-2: Taking Care Of Myself, on page 187.

Think about the impact of these stresses and how you currently handle them. What are you doing to minimize the impact of these stresses on your time, your happiness, and your life in general?

List how you currently handle these stresses in the second column of Worksheet 13-2.

Using the 0-10 scale, mark how satisfied you are with your current coping in the third column.

What other strengths, resources, positives, and skills can you use to avoid, minimize, or better cope with these stresses? How can you draw on your positives improve things?

For example, you might ask family to help with bandaging, massage, or donning compression garments. You can use your intelligence to streamline your tasks and simplify your routine. You can turn to websites, support groups, books, and other sources for support and practical tips.

Write down changes that will improve your life or your emotions in the fourth column.

Problematic Stresses

 Sometimes, the other stresses in our present life make it particularly difficult to care well for lymphedema. Take good care of your lymphedema so it does not cause or worsen the other health problems. Do your best to take good care of other health problems to minimize their interference your coping well with lymphedema.

Other Health Conditions

People with lymphedema often have other health conditions as well. Your other health conditions may be a source of stress. These stresses may take several forms:

- Fear of dying or further disability if you are a cancer survivor or have cardiac problems.

- Physical limitations on movement and mobility due to obesity, arthritis, other muscle and joint problems, paralysis, etc.

- Self-management responsibilities for other conditions such as diabetes.

Other health conditions may interact with your lymphedema at a physical level as well. For example, if you are diabetic and your blood sugar is high, your risk of developing a tissue infection is higher than it would be if your diabetes were tightly controlled.

> ## Coping Suggestions:
>
> See **Resources** at the end of this chapter for useful information on Chronic Illness, Eating Disorders and Obesity, and other topics.
>
> Apply the concepts and skills in this book to your other health problems.
>
> Use the tools for Coping With Unavoidable Stress and the other resources in Chapter 16.

Chronic Pain

Chronic pain is not just a physical issue; it is also a psychological stress that can trigger anxiety, depression, and other psychological issues. Some pain medications may affect your mood and your thinking.

> 66   When the cellulitis gets a wild hair and starts acting up my lymphedema goes nuts too. So I get the swelling and the unbearable pain to go with it. Wrapping isn't an option because my leg is so sore and painful that even when the therapist just barely put pressure on it I nearly cried. 99

If you have lymphedema, you may have chronic pain, either from your lymphedema or from other medical conditions. Lymphedema can cause or worsen problems with the bones, joints, ligaments, or tendons. Good lymphedema treatment and self-care can minimize or eliminate this pain. Good pain control makes it easier to care for your lymphedema. Use the coping suggestions on the next page.

Unhealthy Eating Patterns

Eating problems are addressed here for two reasons.

First, problematic eating can cause excess weight. Excess weight worsens lymphedema and can worsen other health problems, such as diabetes or chronic pain.

Second, unhealthy eating patterns can interfere with good lymphedema care. Problematic patterns of eating can interfere with appropriate nutrition. Having unhealthy eating patterns makes it more difficult to overcome

> ### *Coping Suggestions:*
>
> Seek specialty care for chronic pain. Many medical centers have pain programs.
>
> Ask a physical therapist, physiatrist (a rehabilitation doctor), or rehabilitation therapist about specific physical therapy exercises, stretching, and appropriate exercises and strength training.
>
> Practice good posture. Follow good ergonomic guidelines for chairs, workplace, and other areas where you spend time.
>
> Make healthy nutrition choices and follow a healthy lifestyle generally.
>
> Use meditation, mindfulness, relaxation, and/or stress reduction techniques.
>
> Prioritize your goals. Pace yourself. Manage your time.
>
> For more information specifically on chronic pain, see the **Resources** section at the end of this chapter.

emotional challenges because these patterns can worsen depression, lower self-esteem, and disrupt interpersonal relationships.

Here are some warning signs of possible unhealthy eating patterns.

Check any boxes that apply:

☐ Repeatedly (not just occasionally) you eat an unusually large amount of food in a short amount of time.

☐ You feel out of control when you eat.

☐ You try to prevent weight gain by making yourself throw up, by taking laxatives or diuretics, by alternating bingeing with eating too little or fasting, and/or by exercising excessively.

If you checked all three boxes, it is possible that you have what is called *bulimia*. Even if you are not overweight, this eating pattern can be terribly damaging to your health.

If you checked the first two boxes, it is possible that you have what is called *binge eating disorder*. During a binge, you may eat unusually quickly, eat despite not being hungry and/or eat until you feel physically uncomfortable.

You feel out of control while eating and may feel disgusted, embarrassed, depressed, or guilty during or after binges. Binge eating is often associated with obesity.

People with eating disorders often base their entire self-esteem on their weight or body shape. Eating becomes associated with conflict, guilt, shame, and struggle. The purpose of eating—nourishing and maintaining the body's health—gets lost.

Coping Suggestions:

Notice how, when, where, and how much you eat.

Notice how you feel before, during, and after eating.

See "Eating Disorders" in the **Resources** section at the end of this chapter.

Consider seeing a professional who is experienced in **successful** treatment of eating disorders.

Top Priority Problematic Stresses

These lymphedema-related stresses are particularly serious because they make it difficult to find or afford lymphedema treatment. Without treatment, lymphedema worsens.

Problematic Lymphedema-Related Stresses

Normal lymphedema-related stresses occur even when you have treatment resources. If you lack those resources, you face a more difficult problem.

☐ You have no source of lymphedema treatment or self-care products.

☐ You have no health insurance of any kind.

☐ You have no income or financial resources to pay for treatment out-of-pocket.

If you face these stresses, I encourage you to make it a top priority to find someone who can help you. Without treatment, your lymphedema will almost certainly get worse. Keep asking and searching for help and solutions.

Problematic Living Situations

These life stresses, although relatively rare, are so disruptive or dangerous that they may need to be your top priority. Sometimes people live in dangerous or abusive situations. Lymphedema does not necessarily make this more likely, although it may contribute. For example, symptoms may interfere with being able to work and paying for treatment and supplies may use money that could otherwise be spent on finding a safer living situation.

This issue is addressed here primarily because being abused or in danger make it hard to keep yourself physically and emotionally healthy. Here are some warning signals. Are you:

☐ Being verbally abused?

☐ Currently in a dangerous living situation?

☐ Being threatened?

☐ Being physically abused?

☐ Being sexually molested?

If you checked any of the boxes above, treat it as a **RED FLAG**.

Sometimes people are confused about whether they are being abused. If you are unsure, read the paragraphs below. If this applies to you, read the Coping Suggestions that follow.

RED FLAG:

- If someone frequently screams at you or calls you names, you may be being verbally abused.

- If someone throws things at you, causes damage, destroys objects you value (such as photos or mementos), or threatens to hurt you, you may in danger.

- If someone forcibly holds you down, or if they shove, push, slap, punch, hit, or choke you, or if they threaten you or someone you love with weapons, then you are being physically abused and are in danger of being hurt or killed.

Plan how you will safely escape a dangerous situation and how you will keep yourself safe. If you won't do it for your own sake, do it for the sake of those you love.

If there are children who see or hear the abuse, do it for the children's sake. Children who hear or see physical or verbal abuse between their parents are more likely to be violent themselves or to become involved with abusive partners.

If there are no children involved and you won't make yourself safe for your own sake, do it for the sake of the person who is abusing you. People who are abusive are trapped and can be unable or unwilling to change until forced to do so.

People who are abusive are often remorseful and loving afterward. They may plead with you to forgive them and promise it will never happen again. They may threaten to kill themselves if you leave. They may blame you for "causing" them to become angry. They may try to convince you that the abuse is "justified" or may threaten to hurt you or others if you leave.

These patterns of behavior are associated with continued violence and abuse. Each of these patterns is a vicious cycle that can lead to more serious violence. Staying in this cycle harms you and them.

The person who is being abusive to you is has an anger control problem. They may have a drug or alcohol problem. People who are abusive, threatening, or violent need help. They deserve help. You deserve help.

People with anger problems are much more likely to get help if you refuse to stay in a dangerous situation. Get advice and help on how to leave safely. Leaving can sometimes trigger violence.

If you love them, the most loving action is to keep yourself safe. Protect them from deliberately or accidentally harming you when angry. Encourage them to get effective treatment by not allowing the cycle of abuse, blame, and forgiveness to continue. Use the coping suggestions on the next page.

Complete Worksheet 13-2 by listing any problematic stresses you identified, such as: other health conditions, chronic pain, problematic eating, problematic lymphedema-related stresses, or a problematic living situation, in column one.

Write down what you do to currently handle these stresses in column two.

> ## Coping Suggestions:
>
> If you, or someone you care about, is in imminent danger, call 911, the police, or hospital emergency now.
>
> The National Domestic Violence Hotline (www.ndvh.org) at 1-800-799-SAFE (1-800-799-7233) is a national toll-free hotline for victims of domestic violence, male or female, and is staffed 24 hours/day. They provide safety planning, information, referrals, and crisis intervention.
>
> Help for elders in abusive situations is available across the country. The National Center on Elder Abuse (www.elderabusecenter.org) provides information for the elderly, caregivers, and victims of domestic violence. They also provide an Eldercare Locator service at 1-800-677-1116.
>
> If you suspect that a child is being abused or neglected, call the Child Protective Services agency in the State in which the abuse occurred. The USA National Child Abuse Hotline can provide referrals at 1-800-422-4453.
>
> Talk to people who can help. This may include: family, social workers, health care professionals, counselors, clergy, therapists, police, shelter staff, or crisis hotline staff.
>
> If you are in an abusive relationship, take action now to make yourself safe.

Using the 0-10 scale, mark how satisfied you are with your current coping in column three.

What strengths, resources, positives, and skills could you explore using? Write down changes that will improve your life and/or your emotions in column four.

Stress and Its Impact on Your Life

In this chapter you have identified the positives in your life and sources of stress whether specifically related to lymphedema or not. Review your answers and what you have learned.

Now turn to Worksheet 14-2: **My Emotional Challenges** on page 201 and complete the line for "Current Stress."

Resources

Lymphedema Information

Living Well With Lymphedema by Ann Ehrlich, Alma Vinje-Harrewijn, PT, CLT and Elizabeth McMahon, PhD. Lymph Notes, 2005.

Lymphedema: A Breast Cancer Patient's Guide To Prevention And Healing by Jeannie Burt and Gwen White. Publishers Group West, 1999.

Coping With Lymphedema by Joan Swirsky and Dianne Nannery. Avery Publishing Group, 1998.

www.LymphNotes.com - an online resource and support group for persons with lymphedema and their family members and for lymphedema therapists. It also provides information about lymphedema, treatment resources, and support groups.

www.lymphnet.org - website of the National Lymphedema Network, a nonprofit organization providing information about lymphedema, treatment resources, and support groups.

Chronic Illness Resources

The Art of Getting Well: Maximizing Health and Well-Being When You Have a Chronic Illness by David Spero. Hunter House Inc., 2002.

The Chronic Illness Workbook: Strategies and Solutions for Taking Back Your Life by Patricia Fennell. New Harbinger Publications, 2001.

Living a Healthy Life with Chronic Conditions: Self-Management of Heart Disease, Arthritis, Diabetes, Asthma, Bronchitis, Emphysema and Others by Kate Lorig, RN, DrPH, Halsted Holman, MD, David Sobel, MD, Diana Laurent, MPH, Virginia Gonzalez, MPH, and Marian Minor, RPT, PhD. Bull Publishing Company, 2000.

Chronic Pain Resources

The Chronic Pain Control Workbook: A Step-By-Step Guide For Coping With And Overcoming Pain, Second Edition by Ellen Mohr Catalano, MA and Kimeron N. Hardin, PhD. New Harbinger Publications, 1996. Note: out of print but available used.

Worksheet 13-2: Taking Care of Myself

Stresses	How I Cope Now	How Satisfied?	Planned Changes

Learning to Master Your Chronic Pain by Robert Jamison, PhD. Professional Resource Press, 1996.

Managing Pain Before It Manages You, Revised Edition by Margaret A. Caudill, MD, PhD. Guilford Press, 2002.

Mayo Clinic on Chronic Pain, Second Edition edited by Jeffrey Rome, MD. Mayo Clinic Health Information, 2002.

Pain Relief!: How To Say "No" To Acute, Chronic, and Cancer Pain by Jane Cowles, PhD. MasterMedia Limited, 1993.

www.painconnection.org - an online educational and support community for persons in pain, their families, and physicians. This website is also listed as www.NationalPainFoundation.org.

Eating Disorders and Obesity

Overcoming Binge Eating by Christopher Fairburn, MD. Guilford, 1995.

Overcoming Bulimia: Your Step-By-Step Guide to Recovery by Randi McCabe, PhD, Traci McFarlane, PhD, and Marion Olmstead, PhD. New Harbinger Publications, 2004.

www.4women.gov - a website about eating patterns, obesity, and women developed by the U. S. Department of Health and Human Services, Office on Women's Health.

Obesity info from US National Institutes of Health health.nih.gov/result.asp/476

Overweight and Obesity information from the US Food and Drug Administration www.fda.gov/oc/opacom/hottopics/obesity.html

Stress

Full Catastrophe Living: Using the Wisdom of Your Body and Mind to Face Stress, Pain, and Illness by John Kabat-Zinn, PhD. Dell Publishing, 1990.

The Relaxation and Stress Reduction Workbook, 5th Ed by Martha Davis, PhD, Elizabeth Eshelman, MSW, and Matthew McKay, PhD. New Harbinger Publications, 2000.

Taking Charge Emotionally

In this section you will:

- Review your reactions to the twelve emotional challenges presented in Section II.

- Set your personal goals for any challenges facing you now.

- Learn about the steps involved in the process of change.

- Create a plan for your top most important challenge(s).

Section IV, Chapters 16 through 19, provides a set of helpful tools for successful change.

Section V, Chapters 20 and 21, will help you maintain your successes.

Chapter 14

Setting Your Goals

Ask yourself what you want to change:

- Do I want to change the way I **think** about lymphedema? How would I rather think?

- Do I want to change my **emotions** and feelings about having lymphedema? Which emotions do I want to change and how do I want to feel?

- Do I want to change **actions** that affect my lymphedema? What do I want to do instead?

Maybe you want to change all three.

Let's start with four overall goals that can serve as general guidelines. Then you will identify your specific, personal goals.

If you have more than one goal, you can focus your efforts on the current most important change. Your answers to the questions and worksheets in previous chapters will guide you.

Overall Emotional Goals

As you set specific goals, think in terms of achieving these four overall goals. You want to:

1. Know what you feel.

2. Know what you can change.

3. Know what you can't change.

4. Minimize your distress.

What do I mean by this? Let's take one at a time.

Goal 1: Know What You Feel

You want to be emotionally alive. You want to feel. You want to be able to identify the emotions you experience.

If you are cut off from your emotions, you are cut off from a vital source of information about what's right or what's wrong in your life. Emotions are important!

Learn what the signs of emotion are for you. Especially notice the personal signals indicating that you are not in touch with an emotion.

What are your personal red flags that something is going on emotionally? Check any signs you have noticed in the past or present:

☐ I start to overeat or I crave certain kinds of food or drink.

☐ I dream more, especially nightmares.

☐ My sleep pattern or energy level changes.

☐ I tense my muscles, clench my teeth, have tension headaches, or notice other signs of muscle tension.

☐ My body reacts with diarrhea, constipation, panic attacks, skin rashes, or other physical changes.

☐ Other signs I have noticed:_____

_____

Coping Suggestions:

When you become aware that you feel an emotion, step back. Observe and reflect.

Identify what you are feeling. Name it.

Quite often, we feel a mix of different, even conflicting, emotions.

A healthy emotional life requires acknowledging the emotions we have, even when they are jumbled together and are uncomfortable, embarrassing, or contradictory.

Pay special attention to whatever triggers distressing or negative emotions.

Goal 2: Know What You Can Change

If you're going to the effort of reading this book, you want your time and effort to do some good. You want to focus on the things that you *can* change. This makes good sense, right? So what *do* you control?

Your Self-Talk

You already know that you don't control your spontaneous thoughts and emotions; however, you do know that you can control your response to these thoughts and feelings.

You can *choose* what to say to yourself. You can *change* what you say to yourself. You can deliberately create and practice different thoughts and a different perspective.

Your Actions

You control your actions. Your actions affect the course and severity of your lymphedema. You control whether you seek out and act on information about the best treatments. You decide whether to follow through on self-care and treatment recommendations.

You choose how you spend your time. You can act in ways that support your emotional and physical health—or that undermine it. You can fill your life with activities that give you feelings of pleasure, accomplishment, and worth.

Your Relationships and Communications

You control whom you ask for emotional and practical support and when you ask them. You control whether or not to speak up. You choose what you say and how you say it.

You decide how to act toward others. You can choose to seek out and spend time with people who treat you well. You can say 'no' to others if saying 'yes' would aggravate your lymphedema or undermine your emotional coping.

Goal 3: Know What You Can't Change

You don't want to waste time or energy on things you can't change. Learn to identify what you *can't* change. Remind yourself that you can't change it. Focus your efforts elsewhere.

You *cannot* change the fact of having lymphedema. You *cannot* change anything about the past.

You *cannot* control which thoughts and feelings pop into your mind. You *cannot* control other people. You might sometimes have some *influence*, but you don't control them.

You are only responsible for those things that you control. You *do not* control your spontaneous thoughts or feelings, but you *do control* what you choose to say to yourself and what you do in response to those thoughts or feelings.

You *do not* control the thoughts, feelings, or actions of other people. You *do not* control their choices. You *do* control what you choose to do in response to their actions.

Goal 4: Minimize Your Distress

Life gives us enough challenges, problems, and tragedies. We don't need to add unnecessary emotional distress as well.

Your job is to bring the distress in your life down to the minimum that life allows. This means you want to minimize your distress about things you cannot change.

Accept whatever negative feelings and thoughts you have as understandable. Then go forward to minimize them in the future.

Question your thoughts and feelings in these ways:

1. *Are these thoughts helping me change a problem?*

2. *Are they effective?*

3. *How do they make me feel, better or worse?*

Since life contains tragedies and unfairness, develop a religious faith or life philosophy that accepts this fact and still gives you the courage to go on. Whatever you, or others, have done in the past, however harmful, is now past. You cannot go back and undo it. All you can do now is choose to go forward.

If your actions have caused harm yourself or others, use the ideas from Chapter 11: Asking "Why?" and Chapter 12: Lessons from Your Past. Keep asking yourself the questions above.

The best way to go forward is to repair what can be repaired or to show from your actions that you have learned and changed. This brings some good from the harm.

If others have harmed you, reflect on the saying, *"Living well is the best revenge."* Change what you can to create good in your life now.

Do You Agree?

Do these four overall goals make sense to you? Do you accept them?

If you do not agree with these overall goals now is a good time to step back and think about your questions, concerns or disagreements. Use Worksheet 14-1 and write them down in the column on the left. Then write down the answers or counter-arguments in the column on the right.

If you do agree with these overall goals, skip to the section "Identifying Your Problem Areas on page 196.

Ready to Change?

If you feel ready and eager to make changes, skip ahead to "Identifying Your Problem Areas."

If you are unsure whether you're ready to make changes, but you are interested in thinking about it:

- Complete this chapter with the understanding that you are not making any commitments. You can just be curious about what you can learn.

- Read Chapter 15: The Five Steps of Change. Pay careful attention to the first two steps in the process of change, this may apply to you.

- After that, you can complete the rest of the book. Or you may decide to reread some of the earlier chapters and think about where you are in the process of change with regard to specific emotional challenges.

If you know are not ready to make any changes at this time:

- Skip to Chapter 15: The Five Steps of Change and read about the process of change. Pay close attention to the information on the first two steps in the process of change, Precontemplation and Contemplation.

- Whenever you feel ready, you can return to this chapter and choose a specific personal goal that is right for you.

- Remember, you are in control. Everything in this book is for you to use in whatever way and at whatever time is right for you.

Identifying Your Problem Areas

Turn to Worksheet 14-2: My Emotional Challenges (on page 201) and review your ratings of the emotional challenges. You completed the columns for each challenge as you were reading the relevant chapter.

- In column one you rated each emotional challenge area for its level of severity, distress, or life impact from 0-10.

- In column two you rated how well you are coping with that emotional challenge.

- In column three you identified red flag situations.

Worksheet 14-1: Reservations about Overall Goals

Questions, Concerns, Disagreements With The Four Overall Goals	Answers Or Counter-Arguments

Setting Your Priorities

The last column in Worksheet 14-2: My Emotional Challenges is "My Priority List". These guidelines may help you set your priorities.

Do You Have Any Red Flags?

Red Flag situations are considered emergencies that could be dangerous and life threatening. If you marked "Yes" to any red flags in the third column, you want to make those challenges your highest priority.

Damaging To Your Lymphedema?

The second highest priority is emotional challenge areas that are damaging you physically. As a result of one (or more) of the challenges, are you:

☐ Not receiving lymphedema treatment?

☐ Not doing, or being unable to effectively do, the self-care steps that are essential to the management of your lymphedema?

☐ Doing things, such as getting sunburned, which make your lymphedema worse?

☐ Not protecting, or being unable to protect, yourself from activities or situations, such as having an injection into affected tissues that could cause lymphedema complications?

☐ Noticing, or being told, that your lymphedema is worsening due to increased swelling, fibrosis, or frequent infections?

If you checked any of these boxes, I urge you to make these challenge(s) your top priority, second only to keeping yourself alive.

Other Ways to Prioritize

While I encourage you to give priority to those challenges that threaten your life or are harming your health, I respect your right to make whatever is the best decision for you at this time.

You have complete freedom to choose which emotional challenge(s) you want to overcome and in what order. It is entirely up to you.

Here are some factors you may want to consider. You could give top priority to a challenge based on *any* of these factors:

- **Readiness**: you feel really ready, prepared, and committed to overcome this challenge.

- **Deadline**: there is a deadline you must meet in dealing with an emotional challenge.

- **Easy**: it would be easy to change and you want to start small with goals that seem doable and add more as you build skill and confidence.

- **Frequency**: this problem happens often.

- **Duration**: it has lasted a long time and isn't getting better or going away.

- **Worsening**: it is getting worse.

- **Distressing**: it causes emotional, or physical, distress.

- **Life impact:** the challenge that has a large impact on your life. It may be restricting your life or interfering with your health, relationships, functioning, or pleasure in life.

- **Hardest**: the challenge that is the most difficult. If you succeed with hard projects, you may prefer to dive in and tackle the biggest problem first, particularly if you are committed to overcome it no matter what.

My Emotional Challenges Worksheet

Complete the right column of Worksheet 14-2 by numbering your priorities using 1 for your top priority.

Your Personal Goals

You have now prioritized the emotional challenges you face. Write your top priority challenges in the first column of Worksheet 14-3: How Will I Know I Have Reached My Goals on page 203.

Be Specific

Successful change is more likely when you know where you're going and when you measure your progress.

Coping Suggestions:

Set goals that are specific.

Set goals that are meaningful.

Set goals that seem achievable.

Set goals that are right for you.

For each of your goals write the average Severity and Coping ratings you would like to achieve in columns two and three of Worksheet 14-3. Of course, your ratings of severity and coping may vary from day to day, or even from hour to hour. Your initial goal is to make them better, on average, than they are now.

Measuring Progress

Frequently, ratings in the columns two and three start out being at opposite ends of the rating scale. In other words, those emotional challenges that rate high in terms of distress and impact on your life get low ratings in terms of your ability to cope with them and vice versa.

You might aim for a *lower* number on the 0-10 rating scale you use to measure the overall severity of distress and life impact that this challenge causes.

Worksheet 14-2: My Emotional Challenges

Emotional Challenge	Severity Rating 0 – 10	Coping Rating 0 – 10	Red Flag? Y/N	My Priorities
Feeling overwhelmed				
Sadness and grieving				
Anger and resentment				
Fear				
Self-protection				
Worry				
Increased body focus				
Self-consciousness				
Others' reactions				
Searching for meaning				
Trauma and core beliefs				
Current stress				

You might aim for a *higher* number on the 0-10 rating scale you use to measure your overall coping with regard to this challenge.

As you learn and practice the skills in this book:

- Your ratings of severity/distress/impact should decrease and

- Your ratings of coping should increase.

How Will You Know When You Reach Your Goals?

What does it mean to overcome an emotional challenge? One definition is that the problem gets much less troublesome—or even goes away altogether—most of the time. The distress or impact rating drops and you feel that this is no longer a troublesome area. You have overcome the challenge.

Sometimes, changing the balance between the severity and coping ratings makes all the difference. An area of emotional challenge may still exist. It may even significantly impact your life in some way. However, if you cope so well that it no longer causes you significant distress, this also is overcoming that challenge.

Overcoming Does Not Require Perfection

If you start to feel overwhelmed or discouraged, remember that we all have some distress in our lives. None of us copes perfectly all the time – and that's okay. You don't have to be perfect.

Life is not perfect, nor does it have to be perfect in order to be satisfying and worthwhile. You do not have to achieve perfection to improve your quality of life. Any change for the better will benefit you.

How I Will Know I Have Reached My Goals Worksheet

The fourth column of Worksheet 14-3 is where you can write other ways you can track your progress. Think about what overcoming each emotional challenge will mean to you. How will you know when you have reached your goal?

What will you do differently? How will your thinking have changed? What emotions will you feel more (or less) and how will you know? Be as specific as possible. Write your answers in the fourth column of Worksheet 14-3.

Worksheet 14-3: How I Will Know I Have Reached My Goals

My Priority List of Challenges	My Goal For Severity Rating	My Goal For Coping Rating	Ways I Will Know I Have Reached My Goal

Here is an example of how to use this worksheet:

> Monique's priorities were overcoming Self-Consciousness and Handling Others' Reactions. She never left the house if she could avoid it because she felt so bad about how she looked and didn't know what she'd tell people. She rated her current severity at 10 and her coping at 2. Her goal was to decrease her sense of the severity to 5 and increase her coping to 6. She figured she would know she'd reached her goal when she went out with her best friend, made eye contact with people again, and had memorized a brief response she would give if asked about the swelling or bandages.
>
> After using the skills in the book, she was delighted with her progress. She had reconnected her friends and was socializing again. She went out shopping during the day and even went clothes shopping. She joined a support group and helped others who were newly diagnosed. She rated the severity of Self-Consciousness at 7, but rated her coping as 8. The severity of Handling Others' Reactions had decreased to 4 and she rated her coping at 8. She was also less anxious and overwhelmed. Since she had noticed that she tends to be sad and want to give up, she decided her next goals would be to work on Feeling Overwhelmed and Sadness and Grieving.

If You Have Several Challenges To Overcome

It is quite common to have more than one challenge to overcome. In fact, it is likely that you may have several challenges to overcome. That's fine.

However you have defined them, begin by tackling your top priorities. But do keep this caution in mind:

> *Select no more than one or two emotional challenges (three at the absolute most! – and that's pushing it) to tackle at once.*

You want your energy, effort, and concentration to be focused so you see your efforts pay off. If you try to do too much, your efforts may be too diffused to get results. It is better to tackle fewer goals at first and to make real progress on them. Then move on to others.

Chapter 15

The Five Steps of Change

In this chapter, you learn that the process of change has five steps. You will identify where you are in the process of making changes. Knowing this, you can tailor your efforts and increase your chance of success.

Where Are You Now?

Pause for a moment and take your bearings. Reflect on what you have learned so far. You have:

- Recognized the specific lymphedema-related emotional challenges you face.

- Identified and prioritized your goals.

Congratulations. You have learned a great deal. Take pride in that.

Simply understanding what is going on and observing it can make a powerful difference in what you think, how you feel, and what you do.

Write down any changes you have already noticed in your thinking, your feelings, or your actions since you have been reading this book. Perhaps you are thinking differently about your situation or problems and are actively considering new solutions. Maybe you are feeling more hopeful, determined, or confident. Possibly you have been taking better care of yourself physically, or communicating more with others, or taking steps to reduce stress in your life.

_____

_____

> ### *Coping Suggestions:*
> Be on the lookout for early signs of change.
>
> Notice what you are doing that is making these changes possible.

Focusing Your Efforts

Review your answers to Worksheet 14-3: How Will I Know I Have Reached My Goals on page 203. Keep these goals in mind as you read.

Remember the closing words from Chapter 14. Select one or two goals. Make reaching them your top priority. As you read this chapter, decide:

- Where you are in the process of each change for your top 1-2 priorities and
- What you need to do at your current step.

As you figure this out, write it down in Worksheet 15-1: My Master Plan, found on page 225. This is your guiding plan.

Update your Master Plan as you progress from one step to the next. Change your Master Plan as you surmount one challenge and turn to another.

The Five Steps of Change

Research has uncovered exciting new information about the process of change. Knowing and applying this information increases your chances of success when you set out to change anything – your thinking, your emotional reactions, or your actions.

There are five predictable stages in making *any change*:

1. Precontemplation
2. Contemplation
3. Preparation
4. Action
5. Maintenance

In other words, change is a *multi-step* process. To succeed at making a change, you must move through every step, even if you do so quickly.

Identifying where you are in the change process will help you change more quickly, easily, and successfully. This is because different types of actions are effective at different stages in the process of change.

Let me repeat that. *"What works at one step along the path to change may not work at another step. Knowing where you are along the path enables you to choose the actions that will best help you achieve your goal."*

As you move forward from one step to the next, refer back to this chapter. Rethink what you need to do and adjust your overall master plan on page 225.

Step One: Precontemplation

The first step is called Precontemplation. This is the *"Problem? What problem?"* or *"If I just close my eyes and pretend it doesn't exist, it will go away"* stage where you are not yet ready to acknowledge the issue or the need to change.

Here are some signs that you may be in the Precontemplation stage. Check the items that apply to you:

☐ People keep telling you there's a problem and you don't want to listen. People who are knowledgeable about lymphedema may talk to you about lymphedema-related problems. Others in your life may talk to you about emotional or interpersonal problems.

☐ You refuse to acknowledge any need for lymphedema precautions.

☐ You avoid medical or lymphedema therapy appointments by missing, forgetting, not scheduling, or being late to them.

☐ You do not follow recommended self-management care at home.

☐ You continue saying or thinking things like *"It is no use. Why bother? Leave me alone."* These attitudes indicate that a normal temporary feeling of being overwhelmed has lingered and turned into problematic avoidance, passivity, or substance abuse as was discussed in Chapter 3: **Feeling Overwhelmed**.

☐ You get angry or make excuses when people point out negative consequences of your behavior.

Did you check any of the boxes? As you read the boxes, did you recognize other, similar signs in your life? If so, you may be in Precontemplation. Recognizing this can be the first step of change.

What You Do at Step One

Being at Step One is like not wanting to repair the roof - even though it leaks in several places and shows signs of major problems. You don't want the expense and inconvenience unless you're convinced there is a good reason. And you don't want to hear bad news. You may deny that there is a problem ('no leaks today') or attribute the problem to something else ('well that kind of rain only happens once in a hundred years').

If you are in Step One, your main action may be to stop, look, and listen. Start by getting information and paying attention to feedback. Then, evaluate your options and the likely outcomes.

Stop, Look, and Listen

What are other people saying about your lymphedema care, about your health and self-care in general, or about how you are emotionally responding to lymphedema? Why might they be saying these things?

_____

_____

Look at Your Options and the Likely Outcomes

What are the advantages of how you currently behave, think, or feel? Are there benefits?

_____

What will you lose or miss if you change how you feel, think, or act?

_____

What are the disadvantages of handling things the way you do now? What is it costing you? Are you doing things in a way that feels easier in the short-term but will cost you more in the long run?

Following a self-care program reduces lymphedema. What would fewer lymphedema symptoms mean for you?

Deliberately changing your thinking and actions has many benefits: For example, it:

- Reduces distressing emotions
- Increases self-confidence
- Increases your skill in handling emotional challenges generally
- Improves relationships with others
- Reduces stress
- Increases happiness
- Improves quality of life

What would changes like that mean for you? How do you feel about where you are now and how you are handling your emotions?

Think about the ways you could feel better, physically or emotionally. What rewards would that bring you? What differences would it make for you personally?

Think about changes you could make:

- What one thing would you like to change?

- What one action are you willing to take to start the process of change?

- What are the reasons for starting this change?

Readiness

On a scale of 0 to 10, how important is it for you to make this change right now? _____

What makes you choose that number rather than a lower rating?

_____

On a scale of 0 to 10, how confident are you that you can make this change if you choose to? _____

What makes you choose that number rather than a lower rating?

_____

If You're Not Ready to Change

If your ratings for readiness and confidence are 3 or less, you are probably not ready to change at this time. Continue to evaluate the pros and cons of the status quo versus changing.

Evaluate The Benefits

Consider what good things a change could bring. Get more information about the benefits of changing.

What are more reasons to change? What would make it more important for you to change? What would make you more confident that you can change?

_____

Look Ahead

What is the best possible outcome if you don't change?

_____

What's the worst possible outcome if you don't change?

_____

What's the best possible outcome if you do change?

_____

What's the worst possible outcome if you do change?

_____

How could you avoid or lessen the inconveniences or disadvantages of change? What would make changing easier?

_____

Step Two: Contemplation

The second step is called Contemplation. This is the *"Maybe how I've been handling things isn't so good. Maybe there's a better way"* stage where you are starting to think about and consider changing.

Here are some signs that you may be in the Contemplation stage. Check the ones that apply to you:

☐ You have been thinking about something you might want to change even though you haven't made any specific decision.

☐ You're having thoughts such as, *"I don't like how I'm feeling"* or *"I'm not happy with how things are."*

☐ You are tired of being scared, depressed, angry, alone, passive, stressed, or limited in your life because of lymphedema.

☐ You've heard about lymphedema complications and they make you scared enough to consider starting treatment or changing your current lymphedema care program.

☐ You are increasingly uneasy or uncomfortable about some aspect of your life and future with lymphedema.

☐ You're not happy with how you have been feeling or with your emotional reactions to things.

☐ You're dissatisfied with the results of how you're handling interpersonal situations.

☐ You've found yourself wanting to start making changes in your life as you read this book.

Did you check any of the boxes? As you read the list, did you recognize other, similar signs in your life? If so, you may be in Contemplation – Step Two of change.

Review your ratings of your emotional challenges (on page 201) or redo them now if you think they have changed:

- On a scale of 0 to 10, how important is it for you to make this change right now? _____ What makes you choose that number as opposed to a lower rating? _____

- On a scale of 0 to 10, how confident are you that you can make this change if you choose to? _____
  What makes you choose that number as opposed to a lower rating?

Another indication that you may be in the Contemplation stage is if your ratings for 'how important making this change right now is for you' and 'how confident you are that you can change if you choose to do so' fall in the 4 to 7 range.

What You Do at Step Two

Being at Step Two is like admitting there are serious problems with your roof. You're starting to think you will probably have to do something about them. You're just not sure exactly how much has to be repaired or who will do the repairs. You start to think about how you much you might be able to afford and what the repair would involve.

At Step Two, you want to take two kinds of actions. The first type of action is to explore the pros and cons of changing in more depth. The second type of action is to walk through the change in your imagination.

Explore Pros, Cons, and Feelings in More Depth

Think, talk, or write about your feelings about making a change. What are your goals? What are the benefits? What will be the earliest signs of change?

Imagine and Problem-Solve

Imagine actually making the change. Pay attention to your emotional reactions and look for mixed feelings. Get agreement from your head and your heart. If you have mixed feelings about changing, what would shift the balance in favor of making a change?

_____

_____

_____

Now run through the change in your imagination again. Look for likely difficulties and rough spots. What obstacles will you encounter? What pitfalls are likely? Who will undermine you or criticize? What problems will you need to solve or avoid? What exactly will you do?

_____

_____

_____

Step Three: Preparation

The third step is called Preparation. This is the _"I am really going to do this soon. What do I need in order to change?"_ stage.

Here are some signs that you may be in this stage. Check the ones that apply to you:

☐ You know what you want to change and why.

☐ You have settled your feelings so you feel pretty ready emotionally.

☐ You have identified the likely difficulties so that you can begin to think of ways to solve, avoid, or cope with them.

☐ You are having thoughts such as, _"I really do have to change this." "Things just can't go this way." "I refuse to put up with this any longer."_

If you checked most, or all, of the boxes above, you are probably in Preparation – Step Three of change.

Review your ratings of your emotional challenges (on page 201) or redo them now if you think they have changed:

- On a scale of 0 to 10, how important is it for you to make this change right now? _____
  What makes you choose that number as opposed to a lower rating?

_____

- On a scale of 0 to 10, how confident are you that you can make this change if you choose to? _____
  What makes you choose that number as opposed to a lower rating?

_____

Another indication that you may be in Preparation stage is if your ratings of 'how important making this change right now is for you' and 'how confident you are that you can change if you choose to do so' fall in the 7 to 10 range.

What You Do At Step Three

Being at Step Three is like knowing that you are going to have major repairs done soon. You haven't actually begun, but you have made your decision. You are getting ready. You get suggestions from people who have had roof and gutter repairs. You find information about contractors. You call for estimates. You tell your friends and neighbors. You prepare.

At Step Three, you take three types of actions:

- You plan and think about how to carry out your decision.

- You gather what you need: people, materials, information, etc.

- You make a public commitment.

Plan and Think

Do what works for you. When you successfully made changes in the past, what did you do? What worked for you? How can this knowledge about past changes help you make this change?

_____

_____

Gather What You Need

Find people who will help you change. Build a support network. People can help in concrete, practical ways, can give guidance or advice, or can offer emotional support and encouragement.

Figure out what you need. Collect the materials or equipment you need.

List your questions. Get whatever information you need. Find sources of answers and skills. Read relevant books, websites, articles, etc.

Write down what exactly you are going to do and who will help you—in what ways.

_____

_____

Make a Public Commitment

Go public with your commitment to change. I'm not saying you have to tell everyone. You get to choose whom you will tell. Only tell people who will help you.

But don't keep a decision to change entirely to yourself. Identify who will help. Enlist them on your side. Problem solve with them.

Identify who will interfere or discourage you. Plan ways to avoid or ignore them. Don't let them derail you.

If you want to change how you deal with your lymphedema, find people who are knowledgeable about lymphedema and who are successful in managing it.

If you want to change your feelings, the most effective way to do this is by changing your thoughts, your actions, or both. Find people who are skillful at managing their thoughts or who are successful at taking effective action.

Who, when, where, and how will you tell about your plan and your commitment to change?

_____

_____

Step Four: Action

The fourth step is called Action. This is the *"I'm taking charge now"* stage. This is the step everyone recognizes as "change."

When you first think of changing something, you may want to jump to this step immediately. Other people may suggest jumping to this step directly. But every previous step must be completed before you get here.

If you are still having mixed feelings, I encourage you to stop and pay attention to this. Review the actions for the earlier steps. They are the foundation for change. You want a firm, solid foundation.

Here are some signs that you may be in the Action stage. Check any that apply to you:

- ☐ You have completed steps 1, 2, and 3.

- ☐ You may already be making changes.

- ☐ You have begun applying Coping Suggestions from earlier chapters.

- ☐ If you have already read Chapters 18-20 and are rereading this chapter, you are using several of the all-purpose skills.

Review your ratings of your emotional challenges (on page 201) or redo them now if you think they have changed:

- On a scale of 0 to 10, how important is it for you to make this change right now? _____ What makes you choose that number as opposed to a lower rating? _____

- On a scale of 0 to 10, how confident are you that you can make this change if you choose to? _____ What makes you choose that number as opposed to a lower rating? _____

Another indication that you are in Action stage is if your ratings of 'how important making this change right now is for you' and 'how confident you are that you can change if you choose to do so' are each 7 or higher.

What You Do At Step Four

If being at Step Three is like knowing that repairs have to start soon then being at Step Four is actually signing the contract with the roofer, moving things out of the way, and having the roof replaced. You may not have a new roof yet, but you are actively working toward it.

At Step Four, you take four types of actions:

- You make changes, selecting and using helpful skills.
- You monitor your change.
- You praise and reward yourself.
- You use your support network.

Deliberately Take Action and Use Specific Skills

If you are in this stage, you are making changes right now. Are you using ideas from the Coping Suggestions throughout the book? What changes have you made or are you in the midst of making?

As you continue to read, which specific skills that you learn are you using? Many of the Thinking Skills in Chapter 16 and the Action Skills in Chapter 17 will be helpful.

_____

_____

_____

_____

_____

Track and Acknowledge Progress toward Your Goal(s)

Acknowledge every action you take. Track even small positive changes and their rewards. Periodically review Worksheet 14-3: How Will I Know I Have Reached My Goals on page 203.

Watch your ratings change. How else will you monitor change?

_____

_____

Praise and Reward Your Efforts

Generously praise yourself. Reward yourself. Actively enjoy the positive results of your efforts. Notice your efforts and praise them even when they haven't yet paid off in results.

Specifically how are your efforts rewarded? In what ways or with what words do you praise yourself? If you have trouble praising or rewarding yourself, some of the Thinking Skills in Chapter 18 may be particularly useful as well as some of the Action Skills in Chapter 19.

_____

_____

Support Change

Use the information, the materials, and the people you found in the Preparation stage. In what ways can you make changing as easy as possible? How can you make using new skills a habitual part of your day or your life?

_____

_____

Keep using your support network. Keep looking for role models and asking questions. Learn from others' successes and from your own. Help others (and yourself) by sharing your successes.

Who supports your change? Who constitutes your support network? Do you need to speak up more? If you need to reach out to others, verbally or non verbally, the Communication Skills in Chapter 18 may be useful.

_____

_____

Step Five: Maintenance

Congratulations! You have achieved your goal.

So what's left? Isn't the process of change over once we have changed? Isn't that what change means?

Well, not quite. There is a final step in the process of change.

The fifth step is called Maintenance. This is the *"You mean I have to keep this up indefinitely?! This is getting BO-O-O-R-R-R-RING!"* stage.

Here are some signs that you may be in the Maintenance stage. Check those that apply to you:

☐ You have achieved your goal. You have changed your thinking, your actions, and/or your relationships. You have successfully overcome the emotional challenge(s) lymphedema brought to you.

☐ The novelty has worn off. The thrill is gone. It is less of a challenge and more of a routine.

☐ Others begin to take your changes for granted. Perhaps they no longer offer praise and support.

☐ Maintaining your gains, either physical or emotional, begins to seem boring.

☐ You yourself begin to take what you have achieved for granted. You are tempted to stop paying attention to or working on your goals.

What You Do At Step Five

Let's continue the metaphor of having your roof repaired. You saw the need for the repairs and prepared for them during the Precontemplation, Contemplation, and Preparation stages. You actually had the work done during the Action stage.

Now the roof is finally completed. The roofers are gone. Maybe the neighbors congratulated you. You are comfortable and dry and you enjoy the results of all your work.

But, as the weeks go by, the memory of your effort and accomplishment fades into the background. People stop noticing or commenting. And yet—the roof still requires upkeep and attention.

You must take care of the roof and gutters in order to keep the benefits and to avoid future problems. You need to protect and maintain the changes you have made.

The goal of Step Five is to make change permanent. You want the changes you have made to become an integral part of your personality and your life. You want the changes in your thinking, your actions, and your communications to become more automatic and habitual.

At Step Five, you take five types of actions:

- You continue to praise and reward yourself.

- You take steps to support and maintain your changes by helping and talking to others.

- You continue to track your changes.

- When you falter or slip back, you are able to identify the problem and resolve it.

- You cycle back through earlier steps in the change process as needed.

The challenge of this stage is to maintain and protect the changes you made and to restart them when you falter. The actions below will help.

Praise and Reward

Congratulate yourself. You deserve a lot of credit for having made changes. You should be justifiably proud. Your efforts have brought you to this step. Maintaining change deserves just as much credit, praise, and acclaim.

What will you say to yourself over the months and years? What words will you use to praise yourself and maintain your motivation? What rewards will you notice? In what ways will you reward your efforts?

_____

_____

Talk to Others

Support and strengthen your skills by helping someone else. Teach them what worked for you. Problem solve with other members of your support network.

Explaining and teaching an idea or skill in this book is one of the best ways to learn it. By talking to others about overcoming these emotional challenges, you deepen your knowledge. You also continue your public commitment to your goals.

How will you do this? With whom will you talk things over?

_____

_____

Continue To Track

Periodically, stop to take inventory. What have you gained? What rewards is it bringing you? Review Worksheet 14-3: How Will I Know I Have Reached My Goals on page 203. What are your current ratings?

Specifically when and how will you track whether you are maintaining your changes? How will you remind yourself? How will you make it easy?

_____

_____

Respond to Warning Signs and Restart Change If You Falter

The whole point of the Maintenance step is that change doesn't automatically maintain itself. As the saying goes, *"Old habits die hard."*

It's a lot easier to catch yourself and restart change in the early stages of backsliding. So watch out for those early warning signals.

Be alert to the first signs of returning problems. Do you skip an exercise or self-care? Do you begin to have thoughts like, *"I'm tired of doing this." "I don't have time. I'll do it later." "Just this once won't make a difference."* Are you feeling more bored, tired, frustrated, resentful, discouraged, uncertain, selfish, guilty, self-conscious, distracted, or so on and slip back into old patterns? Are you acting, thinking, or feeling in old ways?

Now list changes in your thinking, your actions, or your relationships that could indicate that you are faltering in your changes or that you are vulnerable?

What problems or obstacles might derail you? How specifically can you avoid or lessen them? _____

_____

If You Get Derailed, Repeat As Needed

When you do get derailed, what specifically do you do to get back on track? Cycle back through the earlier steps as needed:

- *If the signals of emotional challenges have returned and/or if you have stopped your changed thinking, actions, or communication AND you are denying that this is a problem*, reread the pages on Precontemplation and redo the Step One actions.

- *If you have fallen back into old patterns or are noticing signs that you are coping poorly or are distressed by any of the emotional challenges AND you are uneasy about this*, reread the pages on Contemplation and redo the Step Two actions.

- *If you have fallen back into old patterns or are noticing signs that you are coping poorly or are distressed by any of the emotional challenges AND you know you will need to resume changing, but you aren't quite ready yet*, reread the pages on Preparation and redo the Step Three actions.

- *If you notice early warnings signals or are starting to fall into old patterns or are coping less well or feeling more distress AND you are ready to change*, reread the pages on Action, review and resume the skills from the other chapters that have been helpful, and redo the Step Four actions.

Ed's Story

Ed started out at Step One, Precontemplation. He'd been diagnosed with lymphedema but he told himself the swelling would go away and got angry at his wife when she asked him to see a lymphedema therapist. *"Get off my back!"* he shouted. He didn't notice that he was sleeping less, drinking more, was irritable at work, and had stopped smiling and making jokes. Visits by his grandchildren were no longer enjoyable.

Ed moved into Step Two, Contemplation stage when he found his wife crying one day because she thought he didn't love her any more and was worried that the untreated lymphedema would result in an infection and kill him. Around the same time, his boss told him that customers were complaining about him and his best friend asked him what was wrong. Ed figured something wasn't right and decided to see the lymphedema therapist. *"What the heck,"* he thought. *"It probably can't hurt and at least it's a reason to get away from those lousy customers."*

Ed progressed to Step Three, Preparation, after meeting with the lymphedema therapist and thinking about what his wife, his boss, and his buddy had said. He had not realized that lymphedema could be treated. He felt more hopeful and remembered that, until recently, he had been well-liked at work and happy at home. He got on the Internet and researched lymphedema and depression. *"It was a real eye-opener. I learned a lot."*

In Step Four, the Action stage, Ed kept his lymphedema appointments and began self-management. He increased his exercise and started doing things with his wife again. He cut down on the alcohol, and began opening up to loved ones and friends about how down and scared he had felt. The difference is remarkable. *"I like work and dealing with the customers again. My boss says 'the old Ed' is back. The swelling's controlled. And I'm having a great time with the grandkids. It's like that gray cloud over my head lifted."*

Ed is now at Step Five, the Maintenance stage. He handles stresses and problems as they arise and keeps himself motivated. *"Now when I get ticked off, I stop and ask myself what's really bugging me and then I deal with it. Sure I have to take precautions* [to prevent infection and swelling], *but hey, it's worth it. And I know what to do if there is a problem."*

Your Master Plan: Goals, Steps, and Types of Actions

Use what you have learned to complete Worksheet 15-1: My Master Plan.

List your top one or two 2 goals using the information from Worksheet 14-3: How Will I Know I Have Reached My Goals on page 203.

Estimate which step of change you are on now in the process of reaching each goal.

Write in the actions that are appropriate for your current step of change.

Using Your Master Plan

Chapters 16, 17, and 18 provide many tools for changing. Your Master Plan helps you choose which tools are right for the task at your stage of change.

Choose actions that will move you forward in the change process. Move from one step to the next until you have reached your goal. Use your Master Plan to guide you in selecting specific skills.

Worksheet 15-1: My Master Plan

My Top Priority Goals	I'm At Step:_	Actions For This Step

Resources

Changing For Good: A Revolutionary Six-Stage Program for Overcoming Bad Habits and Moving Your Life Positively by John Norcross, PhD, and Carlo DiClemente, PhD. Perennial Publishers, 1995.

Section **IV:**

Tools for Change

This section provides tools that you can use to change and overcome any emotional challenge. These tools are grouped into:

- Thinking skills for changing how you view challenges, your self-talk, core beliefs, etc.

- Action skills for changing what you do, or your behavior.

- Communication skills to help you deal with other people.

- Professional help, if you need assistance from an expert.

In Section V you will learn how to maintain your changes.

Chapter **16:**
Thinking Skills

This chapter introduces thinking skills that you can use to change your self-talk and actions. Why focus on self-talk? Because it is ever present, extremely powerful, and you can change it.

The Power of Self-Talk

In Chapter 1, I mentioned the powerful impact of thoughts and self-talk. What we tell ourselves affects how we feel emotionally. It can affect how we feel physically. It affects what we do.

Let's quickly review some key points:

- **Dwelling on negatives makes you feel bad.** If you repeatedly tell yourself that you're hopeless, ugly, stupid, or repulsive, you are not going to feel hopeful, encouraged, and confident. Your self-talk affects your feelings.

- **Your body reacts to your thoughts.** If you repeatedly focus on your stresses, your burdens, and unpleasant sensations in your body, you are more likely to have headaches, fatigue, and discomfort. Your thoughts affect your physical sensations.

- **You act based on what you think is true.** If you repeatedly tell yourself that things are hopeless, you probably won't even try and you will definitely have trouble persevering in the face of temporary difficulties. Your thinking affects your actions.

Changing Your Thinking

When I talk about changing your thinking, I mean changing what you say to yourself in response to those thoughts that spontaneously pop into your mind. As a thinking being, you always have thoughts running through your mind.

- Some thoughts pop up automatically and spontaneously, without effort. Other thoughts are more active, conscious, and deliberate.

- Thoughts that match your emotions at the moment will come to you automatically. Thinking something that goes against how you feel at the time takes more effort.

- Spontaneous thoughts may be realistic or they may be distorted. They may be helpful or they may be unhelpful.

- You will obviously get better results if your thoughts are realistic and helpful. You can actively work to make your thoughts realistic and helpful. This chapter tells you how.

- Some information will be general. Some will be very specific. Try the various techniques to find which work best for you.

Compassion, Curiosity, and Realistic Optimism

Developing an approach to life based on compassion, curiosity, and realistic optimism will serve you well. Use the ideas below to develop and strengthen this state of mind as you deal with yourself and other people, as you deal with lymphedema, and as you deal with life.

Support Change

Talk to yourself with compassion, with courage, and with confidence. Emphasize every step you take. Praise yourself for what you try.

Track your progress. Celebrate your gains with small rewards. Accept that you will have a learning curve with ups and downs. Notice each small sign of progress.

If you haven't already noted signs of your progress by this point, do so now.

What words will you use to praise yourself?

_____

How will you monitor and track your progress?

_____

How will you reward yourself for your progress?

_____

_____

Learn From Everything

Focus on the positives. Do more of what works.

Problem-solve the negatives. Learn from what doesn't work.

Whenever you can, make the path to change smoother. Look for obstacles in your way. Avoid or minimize them if you can. Put your head down and get through them if you have no other choice.

What are the obstacles to achieving your goals?

_____

_____

Which of these obstacles can you eliminate or avoid? How?

_____

_____

Which obstacles can you make smaller or easier? How?

_____

_____

Which obstacles are best managed by just biting the bullet and tackling them?

_____

_____

You Don't Have To Reach Perfection

Achieving your goals and overcoming your challenges does not require perfection.

Many of us face some of the same issues repeatedly. We have the choice of being either in a rut or on an upward spiral.

You know you are in a rut when:

> You keep encountering a familiar problem. You keep doing the same thing, while wishing the outcome were different. You react in the same way. You get the same unsatisfactory results. Nothing changes in a positive way. Same problem; same response; same results.

You know you are on an upward spiral when:

> You may still encounter the same problem, but with a difference. Now, each time you again encounter the problem, you learn something new or your response changes. Maybe your reaction is less intense, less distressing, or lasts for a shorter period of time. Maybe you cope better. Maybe you think about it differently. You grow in insight, wisdom, or coping.

> Once you get out of a runt and into an upward spiral, each time you handle a repeating problem or familiar challenge, your knowledge and skill increases. The problem becomes less disruptive and distressing. You become happier.

Use Optimistic Thinking

Psychologist Martin Seligman has spent much of his career studying positive psychology. Positive psychology emphasizes what people do right.

He found that people who use what he named optimistic thinking tend to overcome life's difficulties. They are also much less likely to become depressed. The ideas below are based on his research.

I am not telling you to adopt a mindless, unrealistic "*What, me worry?*" type of optimism. In this context, the term "optimistic thinking" is defined by scientific research and means something very specific.

Life is complex. Every person and situation has many aspects. You have some choice about which of the various aspects of any reality you choose to emphasize. The aspects you emphasize powerfully influence your thoughts, feelings, and actions.

People who use optimistic thinking selectively focus on:

- Aspects that are changeable
- Specifics in the situation
- Personal contributions to success

Emphasize What is Changeable

Focus on what is *changeable*. Even when you can't change the situation, you can change your thinking about it.

> **Pessimistic thinking** would say, *"Since I'm stuck with lymphedema, it's hopeless and there's nothing I can do. Since there's no cure, I will always feel unhappy, anxious, self-conscious, self-pitying, and hopeless."*

> **Optimistic thinking** would say, *"Treatment and self-care can help. People with all kinds of chronic, and even fatal, illnesses find ways they can make a difference and have times to cherish. I can change my reaction to lymphedema."*

Home in on the Specifics

Focus on the *specifics* of a problem or situation. If you think about a problem in a vague, abstract, global way, it can seem impossible. Look at specific aspects and facts. When you have a mountain to climb, you don't focus on the peak, you focus on the next two steps.

> **Pessimistic thinking** would say, *"This is all just a huge mess."*

> **Optimistic thinking** would say, *"What specific information do I need? I will set a specific priority. I will take one step."*

Focus on Your Contribution to Success

Focus on the ways in which *you* contribute to success. Take responsibility for your contributions. For every positive change, actively look for what you did that helped make it possible.

Pessimistic thinking would say, *"It's all my fault that I have this problem. I'm sick and neurotic. Sure I feel better sometimes, but that's just a fluke or it's because of what someone else did."*

Optimistic thinking would say, *"There are lots of ways that I contribute to improvements in my lymphedema and in my mood. I complete insurance paperwork, keep appointments, do self-care, ask questions, seek support, get information, talk to friends, etc. Problems happen to everyone. Challenges are just a part of life. I get full credit for my efforts to deal with them."*

Practice Optimistic Thinking

Think about your area of challenge using the three principles of optimistic thinking (what can you change, what are the specifics, and how can your actions contribute to success):

_____

_____

Broaden Your Perspective

At times, the key to shifting your thinking is to change your perspective. Sometimes you need to see a problem from a different point of view. Or examine the problem from a different perspective. Or step back and look at it in a larger context. Here are some ways to do this.

Put Lymphedema in Its Place

Broaden your perspective on lymphedema. Look at it in the larger context of you and your life. Put the lymphedema firmly in its place.

Lymphedema is only part of you. It is not all of you. You are more than your lymphedema. You are more than your body.

You are your memories and your knowledge. You are your creativity and your talents. You are your potential. You are your connections with others, your spirit, your faith, your will. Widen your focus to see all of you. If you have trouble seeing yourself in this larger perspective, you might ask trusted friends or loved ones for their perspective on you.

Write down any other statements that help you to put lymphedema in its place.

_____

_____

When You Are Upset with Another Person

Look at things from different perspectives when you are in conflict or are upset with another person. Use questions such as these to help you switch perspective.

Ask yourself:

- What are two or three more positive explanations of their actions?

- How else could I account for what they are saying or doing that would lessen my distress?

- How might they be seeing the situation that would explain what they feel or think?

- How do things look from *their* perspective?

- What factors might be influencing them that are out of their control?

- If you are angry with them, ask, *"What fears or concerns could be triggering my anger?"*

- If they are angry with you, ask, *"What fears or concerns could be triggering their anger?"*

After you give these factors due consideration, notice how your thoughts and emotions can change. They may deepen or soften, becoming richer, more helpful, or less upsetting.

If you are upset with someone, write your answers to these questions now. Notice the resulting changes in your thoughts and/or feelings.

_____

_____

_____

When You Are Upset With Yourself

Our immediate reactions are not always our wisest. We don't always treat ourselves well, especially when we are upset. In fact, we are often harsher on ourselves than we are on others. Frequently, we tap into more wisdom when we give advice to others—or when we have time to reflect.

You have probably noticed that your immediate conclusion about how important something is often changes over time. It can help to change perspectives when you are upset with yourself.

If you are upset with yourself, answer the following questions:

- *"What would I tell my best friend or child if she/he faced the same situation and was thinking this way?"*

- *"What would a wise, loving, nurturing parent or mentor say to me?"*

- *"If I were at the end of my life looking back to today, what advice would I give myself?"*

- *"How will I think about this at the end of my life, as opposed to now?"*

- *"How important is this in the larger picture of things?"*

- *"How can I think about it to give myself strength and wisdom?"*

If you are upset with yourself about something, write your answers to these questions now. Notice how your thoughts and/or feelings change based on these answers.

Ask the "Three Ways" Questions

We are not born with any guarantees. We don't have a contract that says our lives will be easy or fair. We are given life and the chance to make the best of it.

Avoid the trap of comparing the present to an ideal. If you expect or demand that the reality of life should match your ideal vision, you will surely be dissatisfied. You will focus on the ways that reality falls short.

When you are distressed by something, expand and change your perspective by answering the "three ways" questions. These questions help you put whatever has happened in a larger context. Step back and consider the alternatives.

Think of three ways the situation could be (or could have been) better than it is (or was). Be specific and vivid.

1. _____

2. _____

3. _____

Then, think of three ways the situation could be *much worse* than it actually is (or was).

1. _____

2. _____

3. _____

For example, your situation could be better if: 1) you didn't have lymphedema, 2) there was a cure for lymphedema, or 3) there was no risk of infection.

Your situation could be much worse if: 1) lymphedema was fatal, 2) there was no treatment for lymphedema or for infection, or 3) you were illiterate and homeless.

Tough-Minded Pragmatism

You may have encountered people who take one of two extreme approaches to life. At one extreme are those who think you should always be cheery and hopeful in every situation, no matter what. At the other extreme are those who advise you to always expect the worst.

It seems to me that the middle ground is a stance that I think of as tough-minded pragmatism. *Pragmatism* is a practical approach to problems. The next few specific skills can help you develop this attitude.

What Can't You Change?

You can't change what has happened in the past. You can't change the fact that you have lymphedema. You can't change that there is no cure for lymphedema at this time.

You can't change that, to some extent, your lymphedema may fluctuate unpredictably. You can't change the fact that how you care for yourself can make your lymphedema better or worse.

List what you can't change.

_____

_____

Resolve not to waste time on things you can't change.

What Can You Change?

You have two jobs when you have lymphedema. One is physical and one is psychological.

Your first job is to do everything you can to minimize lymphedema symptoms and to slow, or prevent, complications. If you don't do this, who will?

Your second job is to not add avoidable emotional distress on top of the physical distress of lymphedema. Life has already given you a distressing problem. You don't need to do and say things that will make you feel worse!

Think about these ideas. Select thinking skills that help you achieve your top priority goals.

If you wish, take a moment to review worksheets 14-2 on page 201 and 15-1 on page 225 where you identified and prioritized your goals. This guides your efforts.

Face Ugly Facts Head-On

Pay attention to reality.

To use a metaphor, ignoring the fact that you've fallen into a pit doesn't get you out of it. If you're in a pit, you have to acknowledge it. You can't just pretend everything's fine.

You have to pay close attention to the pit. By noticing, you can determine how far you have to climb, what sequence of handholds will get you out, what tools could help, and what preparatory work needs to be done.

Get the facts. If the facts are ugly, face them head-on. Even ugly facts can be coped with, but only if you face them and actively problem-solve.

If there are some ugly facts lurking in the background that you have been avoiding, denying, minimizing, or procrastinating dealing with, list them now:

_____

_____

_____

AFOG

I love this phrase. AFOG stands for *"Another Fabulous (depending on how you want to translate the 'F-word' in the phrase!) Opportunity for Growth."*

Practice AFOG thinking. Treat every challenge as an opportunity to learn and grow. You may not like or enjoy it, but keep reminding yourself that every challenge is **A**nother **F**abulous **O**pportunity for **G**rowth.

List the AFOG's currently in your life in the left column of worksheet 16-1.

In the right column, list how you might grow, what you might learn, or other benefits you could gain from each opportunity.

Here is an example:

"Fabulous" Opportunities for Growth	Benefits To Be Gained
Feel claustrophobic but I have to wrap and wear compression garments	*I can overcome my claustrophobia, learn to deal with fears, develop skills and courage.*
Have lymphedema and hate it	*Learn and help others with this condition. Develop supportive relationships. Evaluate what's really important to me.*

Motivate Yourself

Think about your reasons to change. Do you like where you are and what your future looks like? What are your reasons to work on feeling better? What thoughts motivate you?

Dwell on the ideas that motivate you. Deliberately repeat specific motivating thoughts.

You can write specific thoughts to dwell on and repeat to yourself.

_____

_____

_____

If you are not very motivated to reach your goals, review the information in Chapter 15 about the early steps in the stages of change.

Coping With Unavoidable Distress

Despite our best efforts, the inescapable fact is that we will all experience negative emotions at times. Naturally we feel bad when bad things happen.

Keeping negative emotions bottled up and boiling inside is not a healthy strategy. Nor is it healthy to pretend that you simply do not feel negative emotions. Here are some skills to use when you feel bad.

Worksheet 16-1: AFOGs

Benefits To Be Gained											
"Fabulous" Opportunities for Growth											

Express Distress Safely

Sometimes the most helpful thing you can do is to give distressing thoughts a safe channel of expression. The emphasis here is on deliberately choosing how and when you express your feelings so they do not harm you or anyone else.

Letting feelings out safely can relieve some of the internal pressure of trying to keep them bottled up inside. Paradoxically, sometimes just expressing upsetting thoughts gives us some relief from them.

Expressing your thoughts also helps you sort out what you're dealing with so you can figure out what to do. (Refer back to "Face Ugly Facts Head-On" above.)

It can help to talk out our emotions with another person.

Sometimes, however, we may not have someone available to talk with or others may not be available to listen as much as we need to talk. Here are two additional safe ways to express distress: Write-and-Destroy Writing and Scheduled Worry Time.

Write-And-Destroy Writing

What I call *"write-and-destroy"* writing is a great technique. Sometimes you can't see something differently until you've gotten the unhelpful thinking out of the way first.

So, let it have its say. Pour out on paper all the rage, resentment, self-pity, and hopelessness. Let it go like a volcano erupting. This is a time to let it out.

Think of it as lancing an infected wound. If a wound is infected, covering it up and pretending there's no infection won't help. You have to acknowledge that there's a problem. You have to open the wound and drain out all the nasty, disgusting stuff. Just let it out.

Don't try to be balanced or rational. With this technique, you are not directly working to change your thoughts in this moment; you are accepting them and letting them flow out of you. Then rip up and destroy what you've written so that it will not hurt you or anyone else.

Scheduled Worry Time

If worrying is a problem, schedule a daily worry time. I know this may sound crazy, but give it a good try because it can be very effective. There are two important parts to this procedure. Be sure to do them both.

Part One: Schedule a time each day to write down all your worries.

You may want to spend anywhere from 20 minutes to an hour. You can keep what you have written or throw it away. It doesn't matter. You can schedule your worry time for the same time every day or for different times on different days.

Some people like to do it in the same place every day. This is a good idea with one exception; I don't recommend doing worry time in bed. You want to associate your bed with sleep and sex, not waking and worry.

Pack 24 hours worth of worrying into that worry time. Do nothing but worry during the time. Don't problem-solve. Don't challenge the thoughts (although this may happen automatically). Don't try to be balanced or rational. Just worry. If you get stuck, keep writing your last sentence over and over until you can come up with another worry.

Part Two: After your worry time, stop and turn your attention to something else.

Go on with what you need to do. If you begin to worry during the rest of the 24 hours, briefly stop what you are doing and make a note of the worry. Say to the worry, *"I'll think about you during my worry time."* At your next worry time, keep your promise. Be sure to focus on that worry, as well as any other worries that may arise.

Don't fight the worry. Don't try to make it go away. Don't discuss it or try to rationalize the situation. Simply accept that it is there and make a note to think about it during your worry time. Then do whatever else you need to do, whether or not the worry continues to chatter away.

Accept, Ignore, Distract

Reassure yourself that no one feels good or thinks helpfully at all times. When you have a rough time, accept it and do the best you can at that moment.

While you are working to change your thoughts and feelings, you will not succeed all the time or all at once. Sometimes you need to simply:

- Accept the presence of distressing thoughts or feelings,

- Ignore them, and

- Distract yourself as best you can.

For all of us, there will be times when we are in emotional and/or physical distress. Making a deliberate decision to accept this fact and then doing your best to ignore the distress and distract yourself is sometimes your best option.

Please hear what this is not. This is *not* being afraid to look at upsetting thoughts. This is *not* denying to yourself that you are in distress. This is *not* choosing to do nothing about your distress.

I am talking instead of making a conscious, rational, deliberate, reality-based decision:

- You evaluate your options.

- You are aware of your thoughts, your emotions, and the realities of the situation.

- You keep working to change your situation, thoughts, and/or feelings.

And, in the meantime until things change, you choose to accept distressing thoughts without either acting on them or constantly spending time and energy arguing with them.

You accept that the distress is there. You ignore it as best you can. You distract yourself by immersing yourself in other activities.

Don't Fear Frightening Thoughts

Tolerating distress is essential in overcoming fears. Studies have shown that all of us have frightening thoughts. It is common to have thoughts that are scary or horrifying. Just because you have a horrifying thought does not mean it is true, or that you will act on it.

Accept and ignore it. Go on with your tasks.

Frightening thoughts are more likely when we are under stress. Some people seem genetically more likely to become anxious and afraid.

Chemicals such as alcohol, street drugs, nicotine, caffeine, and certain medications can make us jittery or fearful either immediately or over time. A good example of this is alcohol. Alcohol can calm you down immediately, but may make you more anxious or fearful over the next few days.

If you think you are just over-worrying, use the scheduled worry time.

If you fear there may be some truth to your frightening thoughts, evaluate them.

Distressing Thoughts May Be Wrong

Thoughts can come into our minds automatically. Such thoughts are often credible, convincing, and emotionally powerful. That doesn't make them true.

You can be afraid and be in no danger. You can worry about things even though they won't happen. You can be convinced that you're a hopeless failure or that no one likes you when the opposite is true.

Distressing thoughts can be mistaken. They can come from a misunderstanding. They can stem from past realities that are no longer true.

Don't roll over and automatically believe them or act on them. Fight back!

Here are six specific thinking tools to help you challenge distressing thoughts. I suggest that you try them in the order in which they are presented:

- Watch your language and your self-talk.
- Question distressing, unhelpful thoughts.
- Consider other conclusions and possibilities.
- Remember your ABCDE's and dispute "irrational" thoughts.
- The two-column technique for challenging distressing thoughts.
- The four-column technique for balancing evidence.

If the simpler techniques don't do the trick, move on to the more involved techniques for challenging distressing thoughts.

Watch Your Language

The words you use have impact. Some words have more negative impact than others. For example, compare these two sentences:

☐ *"I hate lymphedema. I can't stand it. Life with lymphedema is intolerable. It is the worst thing in the world."*

☐ *"I really don't like having lymphedema. I wish I didn't have it. Life with lymphedema is challenging. It is really difficult to deal with at times."*

Check the set of sentences that sounds more like your self-talk.

Which set of sentences will help you cope? Which will demoralize you and make you feel worse? Changing your choice of words can reduce the negative impact of your self-talk.

The table on page 247 shows common negative phrases and more positive replacement phrases. Try changing these phrases in your conversations and self-talk.

Write some of your upsetting thoughts about one of your emotional challenges.

_____

_____

_____

Now write the same thoughts, but replace the negative impact words with others that will not cause so much distress.

_____

_____

_____

Question Distressing, Unhelpful Thoughts

Often we accept our distressing thoughts uncritically. Challenge thoughts that are upsetting and not helpful. Talk back to them. Make them prove themselves.

Table 16-1 Positive Replacement Phrases	
Negative, Self-Defeating, Distress-Increasing Phrases	**Positive, Optimistic, Distress-Reducing Phrases**
Can't	Don't want to Prefer not to Choose not to Decide not to It is difficult to
Intolerable Impossible Unbearable Catastrophic Horrible Terrible Miserable	Difficult Challenging Unpleasant Painful Unwanted
Hate Can't stand Can't bear	Dislike Am unhappy about Wish were not so
Useless Worthless Hopeless	Limited Imperfect

Whenever you have a distressing or unhelpful thought, ask yourself these questions:

- Is this thought true?

- Is thinking this helpful?

- How does this thought make me feel?

- Do I want to feel this way?

If the answer to any of these is "No", then actively, deliberately create new thoughts. Test each new thought against the same three questions.

The answer should be "Yes" to each question. If it isn't, change the new thought until the answers are all "Yes."

Practice saying your new alternative thought over and over. At first, the old unhelpful thoughts will seem more natural and true. But if you have succeeded in creating new thoughts that are both accurate and helpful, then the more you practice them, the more believable and spontaneous they should become.

Use Worksheet 16-2: Questioning Thoughts to challenge upsetting thoughts and to test helpful alternative thoughts.

Write negative or distressing thoughts in the first column. Write the answers to the questions in the next four columns.

Then write new, alternative thoughts in the first column. Test these thoughts by writing the answers to the questions in the next four columns.

If the answers are all "Yes," then deliberately practice thinking these new thoughts.

Here is an example:

My Thought	Is this true?	Is thinking this helpful?	How does this thought make me feel?	Do I want to feel this way?
The swelling is ugly.	*Yes*	*No*	*Ugly, Alone, Hopeless*	*No*
Swelling lessens with treatment.	*Yes*	*Yes*	*Hopeful, Determined, More in control*	*Yes*

If you have trouble finding new thoughts that give positive answers to all the questions, use the next several sets of skills.

Consider Other Conclusions

Sometimes we find it difficult to challenge distressing thinking because we simply have never actively considered other possibilities. If you are having trouble creating new, more helpful, alternative thoughts, ask yourself these questions:

• Is this the only conclusion to draw?

• Does everyone else see this the same way?

• How do other people who cope better or are less distressed view it?

Worksheet 16-2: Questioning Thoughts

My Thought	Is this true?	Is thinking this helpful?	How does this thought make me feel?	Do I want to feel this way?

- What facts are not being taken into consideration by this way of thinking and how do they change things?

Take a distressing thought that has been giving you trouble. Ask these questions. Write your answers down here. Or test them out using Worksheet 16-2 on page 249.

_____

_____

_____

Remember Your ABCDE's

How we feel about whatever happens has a lot to do with how we think about it. Albert Ellis, PhD has written many books on challenging and changing your thoughts. He emphasizes the impact of thoughts on our emotions and actions. He also emphasizes that most distressing thoughts are "irrational" and can be challenged and changed.

To help people remember his thought-changing procedure, Dr. Ellis calls it ABCDE:[1]

- **A** stands for "**A**ctivating Events"—whatever triggers your reaction.

- **B** stands for "**B**eliefs"—automatic thoughts about each activating event that lead to emotional distress or unhelpful actions.

- **C** stands for "**C**onsequence or Condition"—this is the emotional distress or unhelpful actions that result from the combination of A and B.

- **D** stands for "**D**isputes or Debates"—questions to challenge, contradict, or disprove the beliefs leading to the unwanted consequence or condition.

- **E** stands for "**E**ffects"—of disputing or debating your original unhelpful beliefs and replacing them with new beliefs, different feelings, and new behaviors.

For detailed instructions, examples, and forms for using this procedure, see **How To Stubbornly Refuse To Make Yourself Miserable About Anything, Yes Anything!** in **Resources**.

Get the Facts

Here are two more techniques you can use to challenge distressing thoughts. These 'column' techniques focus on looking at the facts behind your thoughts.

The Two-Column Technique

Make your fears or distressing thoughts prove themselves. Test them against the facts and see how they actually stack up with the two-column technique.

Use the worksheet below, a piece of paper with a line down the center or, if you are comfortable using a computer, make a table with two columns and multiple rows. Write down each fear or distressing thought in the left column.

Then in the right column, list all the facts that challenge the fear or upsetting thought. If you come up with more upsetting thoughts, add them to the left column. Keep going until you have filled the right side with all the facts that contradict each of your fears.

Also add in the right column any replacement thoughts that come to your mind. These could be more accurate counter-statements to replace the original distressing thoughts or these could be coping statements. These statements should be fact-based and credible to you. Use language that decreases your distress as explained above.

Sometimes friends or family can be sources of facts or new statements. If you go to someone for help, select a person who is trustworthy and supportive and who can be reliable and objective.

Here is an example of this technique:

Distressing Thoughts	Facts Counter-Statements or Coping Statements
No one could ever love me or want me.	*I don't know the future. My family loves me. I have friends.* *People with lymphedema and all kinds of health problems fall in love and marry.*

What do you do after you have the facts? Well, it depends on whether or not the facts agree with your distressing thoughts or contradict them.

When the Facts Agree

When the facts **agree** with your upsetting thoughts, you have a problem in reality. You need a plan to cope with it:

- Change what you can.

- Find a way to accept what you can't change.

- Take action.

When Facts Disagree

When the facts **disagree** with your distressing thoughts:

- Review the facts and new statements over and over.

- Create and carry with you a file card for each fear. Write the fear on one side. Write the new statements on the other.

- Keep rereading your cards. Use them to challenge upsetting thoughts whenever they pop up.

- Add any new facts that you uncover.

- Act on the facts, not your fearful or distressing thoughts.

Here is an example:

The facts *agree* with Maria's upsetting thought that she is going to have lymphedema for the rest of her life unless a cure is found. She has to accept that she has lymphedema and needs to find treatment, begin self-care, and take precautions.

The facts *disagree* with Maria's upsetting thoughts that the swelling will get worse and worse no matter what, that her life is ruined, and that she will always feel miserable.

Worksheet 16-3: The Two-Column Technique

Distressing Thoughts	Facts , Counter-Statements or Coping Statements

The Four-Column Technique

For more complicated or more intensely upsetting thoughts, you may need a more detailed, step-by-step challenging method. The four-column technique is also known as a "thought record." Like the two-column technique, it focuses on getting the facts behind upsetting thoughts but in even more detail.

Write down your upsetting thoughts in the first column of Worksheet 16-4.

Tackle one thought at a time, so that you don't get overwhelmed. Taking just one thought, go to the second column and write down all the evidence that seems to support the upsetting thought. Remember, this column is only for factual evidence, not opinions, beliefs, statements, or feelings. Make the strongest case you can that your upsetting thought is true and accurate. But – don't stop there!

Now, step back and look at the bigger picture. Look at all the evidence and facts. In the third column, write down every bit of evidence that shows that this thought is not 100% guaranteed true.

Go back and forth between the second and third columns until you have written down all the facts and evidence you can put your hands on.

Finally, look at all the evidence and write an alternative, accurate, more balanced thought in the last column:

- **Alternative** means that this thought replaces the original distressing thought.

- **Accurate** means that this thought is based on facts and evidence you have uncovered and written down.

- **Balanced** means that this thought has to take everything you have written down into consideration. It must reflect all the evidence, for and against, the original thought.

Worksheet 16-4: The Four-Column Technique

Upsetting Thought	Evidence That It Is True	Evidence That It Is Not 100% True	Alternative, More Balanced Thought

Here is an example:

Upsetting Thought	Evidence That It Is True	Evidence That It Is Not 100% True	Alternative, More Balanced Thought
"I feel over-whelmed and hopeless. Lymphedema never goes away. I can't do this."	*Lymphedema is chronic. Self-care takes time. I didn't know how to do self-care at first and I'm still clumsy at times.*	*My therapist assures me that treatment helps. My limb measurements are improving. I'm getting better at self-care. I'm learning a lot.*	*Lymphedema is chronic and self-care will be a part of my life from now on, but I'm feeling better and my swelling's less. I can do this and I have people to turn to for help and information.*

When writing your alternative, accurate, more balanced thought, I generally recommend starting with the more negative part first and then stating the more positive. For example, *"I'm still facing my emotional challenges, but I'm learning more skills, and the more I use them, the better I feel."*

Several variations on the thought record have been developed. Read any of the books in the **Resources** section by Dr. David Burns, by Drs. Greenberger and Padesky, and/or by Dr. Lewisohn et al. Each teaches a way to use thought records to challenge upsetting thoughts. These books offer detailed descriptions and instructions. You may prefer one author's style or approach. As always, find and use what works for you.

What If My Thinking Does Not Change?

Sometimes fears or upsetting thoughts go away temporarily in response to these techniques, but keep returning despite getting the facts. What should you do if this seems to be the case?

Have You Identified All the Thoughts?

Your first step is to ask if you have identified all the thoughts. Spend some time doing inner detective work. Try some of the techniques to Express Distress Safely described on page 242.

Have you identified your worst fears? Have you put into words your most upsetting thoughts? Keep asking yourself questions such as:

- *"What's the worst that could happen?"*

- *"What might this mean for or about me or my future? What would be the worst about that?"*

- *"What's my worst nightmare scenario? And then what? And then what?"*

Don't feel that you have to be 'rational' in your answers. Your task here is to bring out into the open all of your worst thoughts and fears, even if they seem completely crazy or you know that they are unlikely. Our emotional brain is not 'rational' and it is your emotional brain that you are trying to communicate with here.

Have You Gotten All the Facts?

Evaluate all your upsetting thoughts even if, on one level, you know they are unlikely or irrational. Get all the facts. Get specifics. Get numbers. Don't just write conclusions. Instead, write the evidence that would lead to a conclusion.

If you don't have all the facts, ask someone. Find an expert, or two, or three. Go to reputable sources. Observe. Get all the facts that are relevant to you, in as much detail as possible.

Are You Facing Uncertainty?

Sometimes getting facts isn't the answer because facts can only give us partial, reasonable certainty. They can't give us a guarantee.

If the thought in your head keeps asking, *"What if....? What if...? Are you sure? How can you be sure?"* and wanting repeated reassurance, you are probably seeking some kind of guarantee or certainty. This you will never receive.

Uncertainty is inevitable in life. You can never be absolutely certain about anything. Confronting, accepting, and tolerating uncertainty is a challenge we each must face. Running from this, rather than accepting it, just decreases your quality of life.

Apply the thinking skills to your desire for certainty. Use them to challenge your thoughts that certainty is possible or that uncertainty is dangerous.

Are You Wrestling With a Core Belief?

Perhaps you are fighting one or more negative "core beliefs." Core beliefs were discussed in Chapter 12: Lessons from Your Past.

To quickly summarize, a **core belief** is a deeply rooted, deeply believed, general statement about yourself, others, the world or life in general. It may seem obviously true to you.

A **negative core belief** will cause a pattern of similar, distressing thoughts to pop up in many different areas of your life. For example *"I'm worthless," "People can't be trusted,"* or *"Nothing works out in life"* are all negative core beliefs.

Since many specific thoughts may spring from the same negative core belief, fighting one thought at a time is like fighting a weed by just cutting off the part above ground. To really get rid of a weed, you have to dig deep and pull out the root; otherwise it sprouts up again and again. In this case, the negative core belief is the root of repeated unhelpful thoughts that show up again and again.

Changing core beliefs takes more work and a slightly different approach than dealing with individual distressing thoughts. To learn more about core beliefs and how to fight them, review Chapter 12 and the books listed in the **Resources** section.

If what you are doing on your own isn't working, consider seeing a licensed mental health professional. For suggestions on how to select an expert, see Chapter 19 Professional Help.

Strengthen the Positives

Most of the skills we've covered in this chapter are for decreasing negatives. Let's look at some ways to increase the positives.

As the old song lyrics put it, *"… You're got to accentuate the positive. Eliminate the negative. And latch on to the affirmative…."*[2]

Positive emotions, such as gratitude, interest, laughter, and love, have beneficial effects.[3] They reduce distress, promote resilience, improve quality of life, and support successful coping.

Ask questions, such as these, that draw your attention to the full range of positive emotions in your life:

- What creates positive emotions for me?

- What am I grateful for?

- What stimulates my interest?

- What makes me laugh?

- Whom do I love?

Add any similar questions that occur to you now:

_____

_____

List your answers to these questions now.

_____

_____

Focus on these things. Think about them. Seek them out. Talk about them.

Feel these positive emotions freely and often. Strengthen them and they will strengthen you in overcoming your challenges and achieving your goals.

Take an Attitude of "Hardiness"

Drs. Maddi and Kobasa studied people in highly stressful situations to identify what was different about those who did better, emotionally and physically.[4] Their research showed that people did better when they faced stress and uncertainty with an attitude of "hardiness" or bravery.

Hardiness is characterized by: commitment, control, and challenge. Let's discuss how to take an attitude of hardiness in your thinking.

Commitment means being curious and actively attentive to what happens to you and in the world around you. Control means believing that you can affect what happens to you. Challenge means focusing on the opportunities for growth that difficult situations offer.

Focus on taking an attitude of hardiness in your thinking and self-talk. Deliberately develop a hardy approach as you think about life and its difficulties.

By that I mean do these three things:

1. Deliberately find or create a meaningful purpose to your life. Be actively curious about what happens to you and to your body.

2. Dwell on the thought that you can influence your surroundings and that you can influence the outcome of events.

3. Remind yourself that you learn and grow from *both* positive and negative life experiences. Stress, uncertainty, and loss are also opportunities.

What is the meaningful purpose of your life? If you don't have one, make a note and address this when you get to Chapter 17: Action Skills.

_____

_____

What words will you use to remind yourself that you influence your surroundings and you can influence the outcome of events?

_____

_____

What can you say to yourself to remember that you can learn and grow from negative as well as positive experiences and to help you keep this attitude?

_____

_____

Use Praise

Have you listened to how people talk to themselves? We can be pretty nasty to ourselves, saying things like, *"I'm so stupid!" "What an idiot." "Well, that was dumb!"* and so on.

Praise yourself for your *efforts*. Don't wait for full success to applaud yourself. Praise yourself each step of the way.

We do this instinctively when we're young. You can see a classic example if you watch children learning to walk. They stand and fall, stand and fall, stand and fall – over and over.

They're excited and thrilled by each tiny, fleeting sign of progress. They are not discouraged by repeated failures. Their excitement keeps them trying and their efforts keep them progressing until they achieve success.

Imagine if toddlers said to themselves *"Forget it! I'm just not a 'walker'. Look at all the times I've fallen. I bet other kids don't have to work like this. If I was going to walk, I'd be walking by now. This is too hard. Face facts. I'm obviously not able to walk. Give it up."*

Listen to yourself. Deliberately practice positive language toward yourself and others. In particular, praise yourself. Praise yourself for every baby step.

Praise yourself for your self-care efforts and your successes. Praise yourself for reading this book and for being willing to take action to improve your emotions and change your thinking.

Right now think about one of your goals. Look back in time. Reflect on the progress you have made so far and praise yourself—right now.

_____

_____

_____

Remember the Bottom Line

Have hope. We are coping beings. You are resilient. Change what you can. Accept what you can't. Roll up your sleeves and get to work.

You can get through this. You can adapt and grow. You can overcome this challenge.

Write or circle the words or phrases that will help you remember these ideas.

_____

_____

Resources

Changing Core Beliefs

Mind Over Mood: Change How You Feel by Changing the Way You Think by Dennis Greenberger, PhD and Christine Padesky, PhD. Guilford Publications, 1995.

Reinventing Your Life: The Breakthrough Program to End Negative Behavior…and Feel Great Again by Jeffrey Young, PhD and Janet Klosko, PhD. Plume Books, 1994.

Changing Distressing Thinking

Mind Over Mood: Change How You Feel by Changing the Way You Think by Dennis Greenberger, PhD and Christine Padesky, PhD. Guilford Publications, 1995.

Reinventing Your Life: The Breakthrough Program to End Negative Behavior…and Feel Great Again by Jeffrey Young, PhD and Janet Klosko, PhD. Plume Books, 1994.

Feeling Good: The New Mood Therapy by David Burns, MD. Avon, 1999.

The Feeling Good Handbook by David Burns, MD. Plume Books, 1999.

Control Your Depression by Peter Lewisohn, PhD, Ricardo Munoz, PhD, Mary Ann Youngren, PhD, and Antonette Zeiss, PhD. Fireside, 1992.

Overcoming Depression: A Step-by-Step Approach to Gaining Control Over Depression 2nd Edition by Paul Gilbert. Oxford University Press, 2001.

How to Stubbornly Refuse to Make Yourself Miserable About Anything – Yes, Anything! by Albert Ellis, PhD. Carol Publishing, 1988.

Express Distress Safely

Writing Out the Storm: Reading and Writing Your Way Through Serious Illness or Injury by Barbara Abercrombie. St. Martin's Griffin, 2002.

Opening Up: The Healing Power of Expressing Emotions by James Pennebaker, PhD. The Guilford Press, 1997.

Writing to Heal: A Guided Journal for Recovering from Trauma and Emotional Upheaval by James Pennebaker, PhD. New Harbinger Publications, 2004.

Hardiness

Resilience at Work: How to Succeed No Matter What Life Throws at You by Salvatore R. Maddi and Deborah M. Khoshaba. American Management Association, 2005.

The Hardy Executive: Health Under Stress by Maddi & Kobasa. Dow Jones-Irwin, 1984.

Optimistic Thinking

Authentic Happiness by Martin Seligman, PhD. Free Press, 2004.

Learned Optimism: How to Change Your Mind and Your Life by Martin Seligman, PhD. Simon and Schuster, 1990.

Notes

1   How to Stubbornly Refuse to Make Yourself Miserable About Anything – Yes, Anything! by Albert Ellis, PhD. Carol Publishing Corporation, 1988.

2   "Ac-Cent-Tchu-Ate The Positive" by Johnny Mercer and Harold Arlen. MPL Communications, Inc., 1944.

3   "Psychological resilience and positive emotional granularity: Examining the benefits of positive emotions on coping and health" by M. M. Tugade, B. L. Fredrickson, and L. F. Barrett. *Journal of Personality*, 2004; 72(6):1161-1190.

4   The Hardy Executive: Health Under Stress by Maddi & Kobasa. Dow Jones-Irwin, 1984.

Chapter 17

Action Skills

Chapter 16 taught thinking skills. Chapter 18 will teach communication skills. This chapter teaches action skills to help you achieve your goals.

The chapter quickly reviews why actions are powerful and how to surmount two common obstacles on the road to change. It presents general principles to guide you in any change. Lastly, it covers actions that will help you surmount your personal lymphedema-related challenges.

Remember, I encourage you to use this book like you would use a cookbook or first aid manual. It is designed to be comprehensive, but I don't want it to be overwhelming.

Find what appeals to you. Pick and choose skills you want to try. Use what works for you.

The Power of Actions

What you do affects how you feel physically and emotionally. It affects how you see and think of yourself. It affects what happens in your life. This is true for everyone. Taking action is taking charge.

Changing your actions is one of the best and most powerful ways to change your thoughts and feelings. So, go ahead. Start to take action. As Will Rogers said, *"Even if you're on the right track, you'll get run over if you just sit there."*[1]

Obstacles to Action

Changing is hard. That's a fact. But certain obstacles can make it harder than it has to be. I'll present those obstacles and then talk about what to do.

One obstacle is thinking that you are at step 4, the Action stage of change, when you're not. When this is the case, you think you're ready before you are. You may be attempting the wrong actions for your step in the change process. If you are trying, but you are not changing, this may be the reason.

Another obstacle to change stems from telling yourself things that are not true. Two common examples are: believing that you have to feel like doing something before you can do it and misusing the word "can't". These are each discussed below.

You Are Not Yet At Step Four

You may *want to be* in the Step 4 Action stage. You may think you *should be* in that step. But if you're not, you're not. And that's just how it is.

- **If you suspect you're at an earlier stage in the process of change,** go back to Chapter 15: Five Steps of Change.

- Choose actions skills from this current chapter that fit *your stage right now—whichever stage that is.*

- Adapt your action skills as you move from step to step in the change process. Eventually you will get to Step 4, Action stage. Meanwhile, work with where you are.

"I Don't Feel Like Doing It"

We generally accept that our thoughts and feelings influence our actions. "*I think I can. I think I can.*" in the popular children's story, **The Little Engine That Could,**[2] may be one of the best-known examples of how self-talk affects actions. It is not as widely known that it works the other way as well.

Many people make the mistake of thinking that they have to first feel differently about something or think differently about it before they can behave differently. Certainly it is easier to act in accord with how we feel and think inside, but *we control our actions*.

We don't stop for red lights and stop signs because we feel like it. We go to work whether or not we want to and we are generally polite to our bosses regardless of how we feel emotionally or what we think about them. People don't do self-care only when they feel like doing it. *We choose how we behave.*

It's not true that emotions and thoughts have to change before behavior changes. Actions don't have to change last. You are in charge of your actions. Choose actions that will help you overcome your emotional challenges.

The act of doing something creates the belief that you *can* do it. Don't wait to "feel" like doing something. Do it first. The feeling and belief will come in time.

"I Can't …"

Sometimes you'll hear yourself (or other people) say things like *"I just can't."* If this happens often, pay attention to this section. You may also want to reread the section in Chapter 16 on Watch Your Language.

Words are powerful. Our brain takes the words we say literally. You program your brain with your words.

When you say you "can't" do something, you may rationally know what you mean is that you do not want to, or do not choose to, or would find it difficult or unpleasant to do. However, the deeper, more primitive level of the brain that deals with emotional reactions takes your words literally. You can really feel as if you "can't" act differently.

Let's take a minute and define "can't." "*Can't*" means that you are completely incapable of doing something, no matter what the circumstances. You can't move your muscles if they are paralyzed. You can't speak Russian if you have never learned it.

Listen whenever you postpone taking a helpful action because you "can't." Unless you are physically or mentally incapacitated, you probably "can."

Does the situation really meet the definition of "can't?" If it doesn't, go ahead and do it. Don't take "can't" for an answer!

Guidelines for Changing

As explained in Chapter 15, you take different actions depending on where you are in the process of change. Here are general guidelines that apply at every step.

Ready, Aim, Act

Decide what you want to change. Be specific when you set a goal.

Make each goal so specific that you will clearly know when you have achieved it. Write down your goal. Take action. If you get stuck, problem-solve.

Don't second-guess yourself or rethink your decision. Move ahead with at least a few of the steps before re-evaluating.

One Step at a Time

Make it easy to change. Break it down into small steps. Make each step small enough that you are sure you can do it.

It doesn't matter how small each step is. It doesn't matter how many steps there are to reach your goal. The most intimidating mountain, the highest stairway, the longest path are all conquerable. All you ever need to do is take that next small step.

Don't worry about how long it will take. That's not your job. Your job is to take the next step.

Use Action to Change Thoughts

Actions can help your thinking change. Decide what you can do that will make it easier to use the new thinking skills you learned in Chapter 17. What can you do so that you change your thoughts?

Here are some possibilities:

☐ If you haven't already done so, complete the worksheets and exercises in Chapter 16.

☐ If communication is a big problem, skip ahead and complete the worksheets and exercises in Chapter 18.

☐ Make cards with key points from your thinking skills worksheets and exercises in Chapter 16. Carry these cards with you, read them and practice your new thoughts.

☐ Post notes to remind you to use new skills.

☐ Keep a journal. Write down what you have learned.

☐ Start every day thinking of your goal for the day.

☐ Start your day imagining specifically how you will use new self-talk and thinking skills. Do it in advance in your mind's eye.

☐ End every day reviewing every action that brought you closer to your day's goal. Write what you learned.

☐ If you wish you had used different self-talk, relive that memory in your mind, but this time imagining yourself using your new thinking skills and feeling and acting differently as a result.

Add any other actions you think of now.

☐ _____

☐ _____

Check off the actions you will take.

Track Your Progress

The act of measuring and tracking enhances change. **Tracking progress is one of your most powerful tools**.

You can choose to measure whatever you want. You can measure your actions. You can measure your changes. You can track your knowledge and what you are learning. Here are some examples.

Measuring Actions

Measure what you do to reach your goal.

You might track:

• The number of times you do a specific exercise in this book.

• The number of times you try a skill from this book.

- The number of times you carry out self-management activities.

- Physical exercise: how many times, for how long, how far, etc.

- Other healthy lifestyle changes.

Measuring Changes

Measure the end result, not the actions you are taking in order to achieve the end result.

You might track:

- Changes in worksheet answers that show the results of using these tools.

- Measurement of lymphedema changes, ex., limb size (as a result of self-care, exercise, and/or lymphedema treatment).

- Measures of your strength (as a result of exercise and healthy lifestyle changes).

- Measures of your mood (as a result of any or all of the above actions).

Measuring Learning

Measure what you learn, such as new knowledge or new skills.

You might track:

- What you have learned each week from your successes

- What you have learned each week from your failures or problems

- Solutions to problems or ways to overcome obstacles

- What you learned from reading, thinking, observing, or from other people

You may have already begun tracking, using ideas or worksheets from earlier chapters. Have you already decided how you will monitor your progress and keep track of what you learn? If not, do it now.

Look at the ideas above. Check off, or write in, what specifically you will measure in order to track your progress.

_____

_____

_____

Use Payoffs

Make it pleasurable to change. Give yourself little rewards at each step. Reward yourself using things like praise, small pleasures, or positive social contact.

Giving yourself positive rewards is a powerful technique. This technique is called "positive" reinforcement. It reinforces your actions by giving you something positive.

Here are some specific payoffs other people have found helpful. While you exercise, think about showing off your progress. Tell people who will praise you about what you have done. Reward yourself by reading something enjoyable. Put money in a "_positive rewards_" jar.

If you haven't already set up a system of rewards, write down now 10 rewards you will give yourself:

1. _____

2. _____

3. _____

4. _____

5. _____

6. _____

7. _____

8. _____

9. _____

10. _____

Use "Negative" Rewards

Sometimes we can reward ourselves by having something *not* happen. This is known as "negative" reinforcement. It can be a confusing concept and it is one that is often misunderstood so let me illustrate it with a personal example.

Most of the time, I really don't like to cook. To help me write this book, my husband offered to cook on those nights when I was busy writing. Not having to do chores was definitely a reward for me.

I was "positively" rewarded by seeing progress made on the book. I was "negatively" rewarded by not having to cook or clean up the kitchen.

Maybe you can arrange a similar "negative" reward for doing your self-management, or exercise, or using the skills from this book. What would be rewarding to you if it did not happen? Sometimes we can reward ourselves by thinking about the complications or arguments we are avoiding by using our skills.

If you are intrigued by this concept and want to try it, write some examples of things that will reward and encourage your efforts by not occurring:

_____

_____

Adapt

For everything you can't do the old way because of the lymphedema, find an alternative:

- Will you be able to do it again if you follow lymphedema self-treatment and your symptoms improve or if you work up to it gradually?

- Can you continue your activity if you take precautions or get assistance?

- Can you change how you do it?

- Can you change where or when or with whom?

- Can you change how long or how vigorously?

There is a saying, *"When one door closes, another door opens."* If one way to meet the challenge doesn't work, try something else. Problem solve. Focus on what you can do. Find alternatives for what you can't do. Change. Adapt.

Adaptations and Alternatives Worksheet

In the first column of worksheet 17-1 on page 275, list the activities that you currently can't do, or can't do in the same way, because of lymphedema.

In the second column, write down what adaptations or alternatives are available to you. Look at the questions above for ideas.

Fake It 'Til You Make It

Think of yourself as balancing on a scale between changing, on one side of the scale, and staying the same, on the other side of the scale. Ask yourself:

- In which direction are my actions tipping the scale?

- If my actions are weighing the scale toward staying the same, rather than changing, what am I willing to change right now?

Throw the weight of your actions onto the side of the scale that tips it toward change. Throughout each day, we have opportunities to make little decisions each of which either maintains our present situation or moves us closer to overcoming our challenges and achieving our goals.

Act as if you have already achieved your goals. As the saying goes, *"Fake it 'til you make it."*

Act as if you have successfully changed your thinking, as if you have successfully changed your feelings, and as if you have already successfully changed your actions. Pretend you've already accomplished the hard work of change and are now in maintenance stage reaping the benefits!

Act as if you have reached your goal. You may be astonished at what a difference this makes.

See Yourself Successful

You can practice new actions ahead of time – in your imagination. This is a flexible technique because you can do it any time you have a few minutes.

This is a powerful technique because anything we vividly imagine has a physical and emotional impact. In other words, our brain and body respond to what we imagine almost as if it is really happening.

Harness this power. Each time that you imagine yourself feeling, thinking, acting, or reacting in a certain way, you make it more likely to actually happen in real life.

You can start and end the day by imagining just exactly how you will act when you are "faking it." Leap forward to the future when you have successfully begun (or finished!) changing.

See yourself acting differently. Or maybe hear yourself acting differently, or feel the actions, or talk yourself through it. What exactly are you doing? How are you successfully handling obstacles?

Be an actor who's rehearsing a role. Then go out onto the stage of your world and give the performance of your life. Fake it 'til you make it.

Act To Overcome Fear

Both thinking *and* acting have to change in order to reduce fear. If you tell yourself you are not afraid of something, but you don't do it, you will not believe in your heart that you *can* do it and your feelings won't change.

Face your fears. Don't avoid. Here are some guidelines for successfully facing a feared situation:

- Face your fear deliberately, repeatedly, and for a prolonged period of time.

- Pay attention to what actually happens when you face your fear. Don't get so caught up in your fear that you forget to notice the facts.

- Stay long enough for your fear to peak and begin to decrease. Don't leave when your fear is rising or is still high. If you do leave, go back as soon as possible.

- More frequent and longer practices are best for overcoming fears.

Fill Your Day with Small Pleasures

Daily contentment depends more on small pleasures than big events. Bring pleasure into your life several times each day.

Worksheet 17-1: Adaptations and Alternatives

Activities Affected By Lymphedema	Adaptations or Alternatives

Identify or create small pleasures you can enjoy on a daily or weekly basis. Use the list below to help you. Pay attention to pleasure in your life. You could track these in your journal or notebook.

Make a list of what you do that you enjoy.

Add to the list all the things you used to do that you enjoyed.

Now add all your ideas about things you think you might enjoy.

_____

_____

_____

Fill Your Day with Mastery or Accomplishment

We feel good about ourselves when we accomplish something that takes effort or when we master a new skill. Deliberately do things that give you a sense of mastery or accomplishment.

These could include learning something, completing a task, doing self-management, or working on overcoming an emotional challenge. Every step toward a goal increases your sense of mastery.

Make a list of every act, large and small, that gives you a sense of mastery of accomplishment.

_____

_____

_____

Fill Your Day with Meaningful Activities

Find activities that are meaningful to you. Find activities that matter.

Don't sit and watch television all day. Passive activities increase depression and deprive you of important exercise.

Don't wait until you want to do it, or until some perfect opportunity falls in your lap, or until you've run out of excuses and mindless distractions. Find meaningful activities now.

Only you know what is meaningful to you. Write your family history. Volunteer to create recordings for the blind. Advocate for causes you believe in. Reach out to others. Create beauty. Do something for those who will come after you.

Do things that are important to you. If your current daily activities are already meaningful, acknowledge this and focus on that aspect of what you are doing.

List the activities that you do now, or that you can start doing, to bring meaning into your life.

_____

_____

_____

Live Your Life with Hardiness

Research by Maddi and Kobasa on hardiness was described in Chapter 16.[3] When facing stress and uncertainty, hardy people emphasized commitment, control, and challenge in their thinking and in their actions. As a result, they were happier and healthier.

Living your life with hardiness means taking actions characterized by commitment, control, and challenge. What does this mean?

Acting with commitment means staying curious and involved. It means actively learning more about improving your emotional and physical health. Control means being willing to act on the belief that you can affect what happens to you. It means taking actions to improve your lymphedema, your happiness, and your life. Challenge means finding and using the opportunities for growth that are presented by difficult situations.

Those with a hardy approach to life do three things:

1. They are actively involved in whatever happens and deliberately find or create a meaningful purpose to their lives.

2. They find ways to influence their surroundings and/or influence the outcome of events.

3. They repeatedly remind themselves that they learn and grow from *both* positive and negative life experiences and take actions based on this belief.

You have just listed meaningful activities in your life. Now ask yourself:

- *"What actions of mine exemplify hardiness?"*

- *"In addition to what I listed above, what else specifically do I do that gives meaningful purpose to my life?"*

- *"How do I, or could I, influence my world?"*

- *"What action(s) am I taking (or could I take) that foster growth?"*

Write your answers here. Act on your answers.

_____

_____

Express Positive Emotions through Actions

You are putting pleasure and meaning into your life. You are changing your thoughts, actions, and feelings. Express your positive emotions through actions.

Share these positive emotions that you have been developing. How many times a day can you express positive emotions? How many different ways can you find?

You can express them in speaking to others. You can write about them to others or in a journal or diary. You can express them through poetry, art, music, or other means.

You can express them nonverbally through your tone and expressions. You can show them through physical gestures to others in hugging, affectionate or grateful touching, or in other ways. You can express them in prayer or other religious or meditative practices.

List the specific ways that you will express your positive emotions through action.

_____

_____

Don't Go It Alone

Surround yourself with others who empathize with your feelings and support your efforts. Find people who support your accomplishments. Let them support your efforts. Let them help you. *"Hardy individuals.... use active coping and social support..."*[4]

You are responsible for taking care of yourself and meeting your challenges, but you don't have to do it alone. Reach out for help until you find it.

Cultivate a support network and actively use it. Take classes. Participate in a chat room. Lymph Notes (www.LymphNotes.com) and NLN (www.lymphnet.org) are reputable websites where you can locate support groups, chat rooms, sources of information and education, and other resources.

Join or start a support group. Attend a therapy group. Become involved in activities through your community center, your religious organization, or your interest groups.

Talk to everyone who could possibly help you or support you. Tell them your goals and what you need. Ask them to help, either by specific actions or giving emotional support. Share your progress.

People differ in the amount and type of help they prefer. Write exactly how you now currently (or will in the future) find and benefit from help.

_____

_____

_____

Take Care of Yourself

The actions below are important for the overall health of your body. Many of them are also significant stress reducers. Chronic stress is associated with chemical actions in the brain and body that seem to be harmful to the body over time.

Take these actions seriously. Build as many of them into your daily life as possible.

Maintain Health

Take care of yourself while you work through your emotional challenges:

- Get an adequate amount of sleep so that you are refreshed.

- Get enough exercise to maintain your health.

- Eat healthfully, get the nutrients you need, and drink enough healthy fluids.

- Maintain your lymphedema self-management routines.

Reduce Stress

Reduce your stress and your reactions to stress.

- A healthy lifestyle, exercise, and good sleep all reduce stress.

- Set realistic priorities and manage your time.

- Delegate where appropriate.

- Problem-solve.

- Take moments of relaxation.

- Connect with your sources of love and inspiration.

- Build stress reducers into your life such as slow deep breathing, yoga, meditation, swimming, massage, exercise, lymphedema massage, etc.

Practice Relaxation and Exercise

Relaxation and exercise help emotionally and physically:

- Yoga, mindfulness, tai chi, and other meditation-based activities can reduce emotional distress and help you cope with difficult times.

- Diaphragmatic breathing (slow deep breathing) and muscle relaxation can help you tolerate fear or other distressing emotions.

- Diaphragmatic breathing (slow deep breathing) helps move the lymph.

- Exercise reduces stress, improves sleep, protects health, and lifts mood.

- Muscle movements move lymph fluid. Walking or water exercises can be both relaxing and invigorating.

Yes, But....

Do you still find yourself procrastinating? Try these techniques.

When One Job Is Hard, Two May Be Easier

You are procrastinating on an important task. You know it is important to you but you're having trouble actually doing it. Here is a trick.

Identify one or two *other* tasks. These should also be important or necessary, but not particularly enjoyable. "Procrastinate" and "avoid" these other tasks by working on the first one.

Take turns procrastinating and avoiding—by moving from one task to the other. This way, you get to avoid, postpone, and procrastinate, while still getting something important done. No matter what you work on, you end up making progress. I used this technique to complete my dissertation in graduate school.

Don't Just Do Something, Stand There!

This technique came from a marvelous little book by Alan Lakein.[5] Everyone procrastinates at times. Sometimes deep inside we know that, by doing anything other than our most important tasks, we are really just wasting time. But keeping busy pushes that awareness away.

Use this technique to interrupt that process. When you realize that you are avoiding one of your most important tasks, immediately stop whatever you are doing. Don't do something else instead. Don't do something distracting, entertaining, or less important. Do nothing. Simply nothing. Truly acknowledge that, by not working on your most important task, you are wasting your time. If you are going to waste time, waste time.

Notice what you are doing. What are you thinking? How are you feeling? Stop and pay attention. This gives you the opportunity to make a thoughtful, aware, conscious decision about how to use your time. Once you have stopped rushing around wasting time and actually stopped to pay attention, you can make a choice.

You can choose to stop procrastinating and go to work on what's most important. You can reorganize your priorities and choose to work on something less important. You can decide to take a deliberate break and return to your important job at a particular time.

The important thing is that *you* are choosing. The purpose of this technique—just like the purpose of this book—is to put you in the driver's seat. After all, it's your life, your time, and your body.

Resources

www.LymphNotes.com an online resource and support group for persons with lymphedema and their family members and for lymphedema therapists. It also provides information about lymphedema, treatment resources, and support groups.

www.lymphnet.org website of the National Lymphedema Network, a nonprofit organization providing information about lymphedema, treatment resources, and support groups.

Notes

1   From www.quotationspage.com "Motivational Quotes of the Day"

2   **The Little Engine That Could** by Watty Piper. Platt & Munk, 1930.

3   **The Hardy Executive: Health Under Stress** by Maddi & Kobasa. Dow Jones-Irwin, 1984.

4   "Loss, Trauma, and Human Resilience: Have We Underestimated the Human Capacity to Thrive after Extremely Aversive Events?" by G. Bonanno. *American Psychologist* January 2004; vol. 59 no. 1: 20-28. (p. 25)

5   **How To Get Control Of Your Time And Your Life** by Alan Lakein. Signet, 1996.

Chapter **18:**

Communication Skills

This chapter teaches communication skills that apply to most situations. It also offers suggestions for special situations. Let's start with the most basic skills.

The Communication Sandwich

If you go to the trouble of communicating something unpleasant or difficult, you want to be heard. You are more likely to be heard if you emphasize the positive at the start and the end of what you say.

Here's a simple suggestion; think of it as a communication sandwich:

- **First,** say something sincerely positive to introduce what you have to say.

- **Then,** offer the more negative, difficult part of the communication.

- **Finish up** with something positive.

You only bring up a problem because you care about the relationship or situation and want to resolve it. You can emphasize the positive reasons for the discussion, the positive aspects of the relationship, and/or the positive goal you want to achieve. The positives have to be something you honestly mean.

Let me give you two examples.

Example One:

> **Situation:** Your spouse is doing more chores around the house now that you have lymphedema and you are unhappy with how the chores are being done.
>
> **Positive:** *"I really appreciate your help with these chores."*
>
> **Negative:** *"At the same time, you do them less often than I would and that's frustrating to me. Things around the house look messy and dirty to my eyes. Would it be possible to do some of the chores more often? Is there a way I can help?"*
>
> **Positive:** *"I see the extra work you do and I want to come up with a solution that we both feel good about. This has been bothering me and I don't want it to be an issue between us because you're the most important person in my life."*

Example Two:

> **Situation:** Your friend has suggested that you go out for a long, vigorous hike in the heat of the day. Your lymphedema therapist has advised you not to do heavy exercise in the heat.
>
> **Positive:** *"I love getting together with you. Thank you for suggesting it."*
>
> **Negative:** *"I'm really uncomfortable exercising vigorously in such hot weather and bright sun."*
>
> **Positive:** *"But I do want to do things with you that we both enjoy. How about if we go for a hike when it's cool, or walk in the air-conditioned mall, or do something else?"*

Use worksheet 18-1 on page 285 to practice your new sandwich making skills.

- Write a brief description of the situation.

- Then fill in your communication sandwich: First a positive, then the negative or problem, and then a positive.

If you remember nothing else about communicating, remember to begin and end with a positive.

Worksheet 18-1: Making a Communication Sandwich

Situation	Positive	Negative	Positive

Five Positives to Every One Negative

Research psychologists John Gottman and colleagues have been studying communication between couples for years.[1] Couples were videotaped as they discuss topics on which they disagree and their communications were evaluated for the number of positives and negatives.

All couples started out deeply in love and began their relationships with commitment, love, and optimism. All couples, happy and unhappy, had disagreements. And, for all couples, the same issues tended to be causes of disagreements.

Despite these similarities, researchers learned to predict with roughly 90% accuracy which couples would remain happy and which would not. How? By evaluating the way they communicated with each other.

Successful couples had at least five positive interactions to every negative interaction. This pattern predicted a lasting, happy marriage. Couples with fewer positives to each negative tended to have unhappy marriages that frequently ended in divorce.

Communication positives are actions such as:

- Nodding, eye contact, smiling, making an empathic face
- Using a tone of voice that is caring, warm, affectionate, concerned, empathic, or happy
- Paying attention
- Leaning toward the other person with open arms and with a relaxed body posture
- Smiling
- Affectionate touching

Communication negatives include:

- Sarcasm
- Angry tone of voice or yelling
- Dismissing what the other person has said
- Belittling or criticizing

- Avoiding eye contact

- Turning away physically

To learn more about communicating in ways that protect your marriage or any other relationship that is important to you, see the books listed under General Communication Skills in the **Resources** section.

Meanwhile, remember the take-home message: 5 to 1. You want at least 5 positive interactions or comments to every 1 negative. (This is a good rule to follow even when talking to yourself!)

Six Basic Communication Skills

The more skills you use, the more effective you'll be. So let's move on to the six all-purpose communication skills. These skills incorporate what you have just learned.

These basic skills apply to most situations. Use them in the order in which they are presented. In different situations, you'll emphasize some skills more than others.

1. Ask and listen.

2. Check what you think you heard.

3. Find something to agree with.

4. Be honest about your contribution to the problem or situation.

5. State your side.

6. Find solutions that work for everyone.

If you have trouble using these skills, turn to **Resources** at the end of this chapter and read one or more of the books under the heading General Communication Skills. You can also improve your communication skills through communication classes, couples counseling, parenting classes, family therapy, or individual psychotherapy.

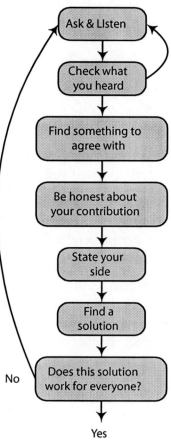

Ask and Listen

Start by asking questions and really listening to the answers. I mean, really listening. Not just sitting there thinking of your comebacks or your reactions.

Listen to the other person. Elicit their concerns and views. Let them feel fully heard and understood.

It can be hard to hear that persons you care about see or feel things differently than you do. You may be tempted to interrupt, to attack, to defend, to explain—anything but listen. But listening is the first step to communicating.

Your most important task right now is to help them express their views and their feelings. This is especially important when you disagree with what they say or feel.

If you don't talk about differences, you can't resolve them. You already know what *you* think and feel. Listen to *them*.

Check What You Think You Heard

Make sure that you accurately heard what the other person said—however wrong you think they are! You do this by restating your understanding of what you believe they think and feel.

Say it from their viewpoint. You are not agreeing or giving in to them. You are verifying that you understood them correctly.

If you don't understand what they are saying, ask a few essential questions and apply your listening skills. If you understand *what* they are saying, but can't comprehend *why* they think it, you may also want to back up to "Ask and Listen."

If *you* think you understand, but *they* feel you don't understand, then you have probably missed something. Cycle back to "Ask and Listen" again. Don't move forward until you get the okay from the other person that you understand what they are thinking and how they are feeling.

Find Something to Agree With

Start by agreeing with everything that you honestly can agree with. Don't lie. But, before you do anything else, after checking that you heard correctly, find things to agree with.

Sometimes you agree with them completely. (That's easy, but it doesn't happen very often.)

What do you do when you are not in complete agreement? Consider these options:

- Can you agree with the facts?

- Can you agree that their emotions are understandable, given what they know or believe to be true?

- Can you agree with part of what they say?

- Can you agree with their goals?

- Can you agree with their values?

Find something with which you can agree. You need to establish a common ground. You want the other person to hear you. Other people usually can't listen until they feel their viewpoint has been heard.

Your job is to convince them that it is safe to talk about uncomfortable feelings. You need to demonstrate through your words, actions, and tone of voice that you can be trusted to treat their needs and feelings with respect—even when you disagree.

Be Honest About Your Contribution

Look for ways in which you contribute to the problem. Here are some ways in which people commonly contribute to problems.

Ask yourself if you do any of these. Check off all that apply to you:

- ☐ Avoid asking about the other person's feelings or viewpoint.

- ☐ Avoid talking about your own feelings or making requests.

- ☐ Make requests in a way that is not direct or respectful.

- ☐ Get angry, impatient, sarcastic, critical, or irritable.

☐ Get upset, tearful, or defensive.

☐ Have trouble negotiating, so instead you attack, try to manipulate, withdraw, or give up.

☐ Agree to do something, but then do not actually follow through.

☐ Make assumptions without stating them or verifying them.

Openly admit these actions. I know this is hard, but think of it as being honest.

Taking responsibility for your role is like putting a deposit in the "trust bank." If the other person can trust you to honestly admit the ways *you* contribute to unresolved problems, they are more likely to listen to ways you think *they* contribute to unresolved problems.

State Your Side

Now state the ways in which you feel and see things differently from the other person. Be just as clear and respectful of *your* concerns and your views as you were of theirs.

Say how you feel and what you want in a way that is as easy as possible for others to understand. Stand your ground. Respect and accept your own feelings as much as theirs.

If the other person finds it hard to listen and accept, repeat the cycle of earlier skills as often as needed: 1) ask and listen; 2) check what you think you heard until you get confirmation; 3) find something in what they said that you agree with; and 4) be honest about any way you contribute to the problem. But eventually get back to standing up for yourself and stating your side.

For a successful negotiation, everyone has to be involved—and that includes you. For a negotiation that improves the relationship and that will stand over time, everyone's feelings and desires need to be accommodated—which leads us to the final skill.

Find Solutions That Work For Everyone

Work together to find solutions. The only rule about solutions is that they have to be at least minimally acceptable to everyone.

Solutions that satisfy only one person won't work. Solutions that don't take reality into account won't work. Solutions where one person isn't honest won't work.

Finding a solution is like planning a car trip when you have two or more drivers sharing the driving. Misunderstandings and disagreements about route and destination have to be worked out. Unless everyone agrees, one driver will go in one direction, while the next may head off in a different direction entirely. Each may believe he is right and blame the other.

You might be able to bully or manipulate your way into an unfair solution, but you'll pay the price. The relationship suffers. No one is happy in the long run. The solution is unlikely to last. The discomfort of honest negotiation pays off. Following these skills is worth the work.

When NOT To Communicate

Consider what is safe to communicate. Do not start difficult discussions if others react with violence or threats of violence. Your job is to stay safe. If someone is threatening or physically harming you at home or work, this is an emergency. Find a way to make your situation safe or to find a safe alternative. Everything else comes second. Sadly, there are times when you have to limit or discontinue contact with another person for your own physical, financial, or emotional safety. Do what you have to do to protect yourself.

Consider what is appropriate to communicate. What you say to family is different from what you tell strangers. How and what you communicate to coworkers may be different from how and what you communicate to your supervisor or boss.

Communicating With Family Members

Your family members are likely dealing with some of the same thoughts and emotional issues you face. They may feel sorrow, grief, guilt, fear, worry, anger, pity, and/or resentment.

They may feel helpless and confused. They may not understand. They may want the problem to disappear. They may treat you as if you are fragile and helpless. They may respond to the pain of difficult emotions by getting angry or withdrawing.

Chapter 22: is addressed specifically to family and friends. Family members may also want to read some or all of the earlier chapters in this book.

Relationships respond to the strain of chronic illness in one of two ways. They get stronger or they get weaker. Something *will* change. You want your actions to help the relationship change for the better.

Review the section on Family in Chapter 10. I also encourage you to read Chapter 22: For Family and Friends because it presents some of these ideas in a slightly different way.

Remember that it is lymphedema with its resultant stresses, challenges, painful feelings, and dilemmas that is the problem. Don't let the problems or disagreements that lymphedema can bring into your life turn you and your family members against one another. They are not the enemy; lymphedema is.

The two of you don't want to face off and fight against each other. You want to side with one another and fight together against the challenges of lymphedema.

Be prepared to be patient. Use all the communication skills and keep using them. Focus on understanding and accepting your family member. Remind yourself that everyone is unique and no one is perfect.

Sometimes there are additional factors to take into account when you communicate with a family member. Memory, concentration, or attention span can be affected by factors such as emotion, psychological problems, medication, medical conditions, or aging.[2]

Make sure you have realistic expectations about what a family member can understand and recall. You may need to adapt your communication style. You may need to leave notes and reminders.

Talking With Children

If you have lymphedema, your children or grandchildren may have questions or concerns. You may want to explain what lymphedema is and how it affects what you can do.

Use the basic communication skills. This is important for two reasons:

- First, these skills will help you communicate more effectively.

- Second, children learn how to communicate and handle conflict by watching the adults around them. Talk with them the way you want them to talk with you.

Review the section on Others' Reactions in Chapter 10 for information on some of the common concerns children may have about your lymphedema.

Adjust what you say to match a child's individual temperament and stage of development. See the section, Your Child Is Unique, in Chapter 23 for more information.

The **Resources** section the end of this chapter includes books about communication skills for parents.

Communicating With Sexual Partners

Sexuality is an emotion-charged area that many of us find difficult to talk about during the best of times Sexuality may be impacted by the original cause of the lymphedema, by lymphedema itself, and/or by the emotional reactions to lymphedema. .

Sexuality Issues

Some of the problems that cause lymphedema can also cause loss of sexual desire, decrease in sexual response, and/or infertility. Talk with your health-care professionals if you suspect this to be the case.

Sexuality can also be impacted by any of the other emotional challenges covered earlier. It is hard to relax and be sexual if you feel anxious, self-conscious, depressed, angry, overwhelmed, traumatized, or stressed. A payoff of handling other emotional problem areas is that you become more likely to enjoy sex.

The more lymphedema symptoms are controlled and the better you feel emotionally, the easier and more satisfying sexual contact can be.

Identify any issues you face currently. Check those that apply to you:

☐ Worrying about your partner's response to the physical signs of lymphedema.

☐ Feeling more self-conscious during foreplay or sex.

☐ Noticing a decrease in sexual desire or responsiveness.

Megan's Story

Megan was fourteen when she developed primary lymphedema in her right foot and leg. With good treatment her lymphedema was under control and she had done well in high school and college. Megan loved children and in college she majored in education. Soon after graduation she met Brad and knew he was "the one." Brad shared these feelings and they began to talk about marriage. This should have been a happy time but Megan was worried. She so much wanted to have children but what about the lymphedema? Would the strain of a pregnancy affect her lymphedema? Since this is an inherited condition, would she pass it on to her children?

Instead of seeking help, or sharing these concerns with Brad, Megan worried in silence. The longer she worried, the darker the picture became in her mind, and the more she pulled away from Brad.

It wasn't long before Brad realized that something was wrong. He knew about Megan's lymphedema and it wasn't a big deal to him so he thought there must be something wrong with their relationship.

Finally he confronted Megan with his concerns and she shared her worries with him. Together they learned all they could about primary lymphedema and any potential difficulties that it might present in raising a family. With this information, they decided that there were no issues that they could not manage together and soon announced their engagement.

Write down any other issues you identify.

_____

_____

You may want to reread the section in Chapter 9: Self-Consciousness on "Normal Self-Consciousness and Sexuality."

If physical intimacy is important to you, actively work to make it happen. When you have a chronic condition, sex may require planning and adaptation.

Use these four suggestions for communicating about sexuality issues:

1. Start with you.

2. Talk with your partner.

3. Discover what works.

4. Focus on pleasure.

Step 1: Start With You

Start with you. Only you know what you feel, emotionally and physically. Only you know what pleases and excites you.

Explore your thoughts and feelings about sex and your body. Ask yourself, *"What needs to change in order for me to enjoy sex? What can I do to make those changes?" "What is my sexual goal?" "What needs to happen to achieve that goal? What ideas do I have"*

Write your answers down here or in a private journal.

_____

_____

_____

Step 2: Talk With Your Partner

Explore your partner's thoughts and feelings about sex. Use the communication skills discussed above.

Begin by understanding the other person's views, feelings, concerns, and hopes. Then share your own feelings with your partner. You can't solve or work around a problem if you don't know it exists. You and your partner have to talk to each other.

Talk about pleasures as well as problems. Let your partner know what feels pleasurable to you. Actively learn what feels pleasurable to him or her.

You must tell or show the other person. The nerves in your body send signals to your brain only, not your partner's. Your partner can't sense what feels good to you—and vice versa.

Step 3: Discover What Works

Problem-solve together. Here are examples of changes that couples have found helpful:

- Change positions. Find positions that are comfortable and don't aggravate the lymphedematous body area. If you are searching for ideas, start with the books under Sexuality in **Resources** at the end of this chapter.

- Spend time preparing for sexual encounters.

- Create and maintain arousal by deliberately focusing on sexually stimulating images or memories.

- Consciously focus on the pleasurable physical sensations, tastes, or scents.

- Spend more time in foreplay.

- Share non-sexual, pleasurable touching.

What are the two of you doing currently? What increases relaxation and pleasure? What blocks or disrupts relaxation and pleasure?

Some couples are comfortable with using lubricants, vibrators, erotica, and/ or sexual toys to increase arousal. Discover what works for the two of you. Write it down here or elsewhere. Then do more of it.

_____

_____

_____

Step 4: Focus on Pleasure

Keep your focus on pleasure, not necessarily orgasm. Sex should be an experience of freely shared pleasure. It is not a performance that will be reviewed and critiqued. It should not be an exam that you, or your body, pass or fail.

Sexual contact should be a process of giving and receiving pleasure. Focus on that experience. Become immersed in the moment. Paradoxically, the more you focus just on the pleasures of the moment, the more aroused you may become.

Do you worry about your partner's response to your body? If so, I have good news for you. The more aroused your partner becomes, the more perfect your body looks to him or her.

Actively use your mind in the service of your sexuality. Use Worksheet 18-2: Focus on Pleasure to help you. Fill out this worksheet on page 299 or copy it and fill it out elsewhere.

Notice what thoughts spontaneously come to your mind during sex. What are you saying to yourself? Write them in the first column.

Then for each thought, write down in the second column whether it increases or decreases sexual pleasure.

For each thought that *decreases* pleasure, decide what you will substitute and focus on instead. Write those in the third column. They may be words, instructions, or sayings. They may be mental pictures or images. They may be memories or fantasies.

Use your mind's incredible ability to imagine, recall, and fantasize. Shared physical intimacy, like shared emotional intimacy, can be deeply healing.

Pregnancy Issues

If you are a couple who is considering having a child, and one or both of you has primary lymphedema, you may want genetic counseling to understand the risks of your child inheriting primary lymphedema. Ask your obstetrician for a referral.

If you are female with lymphedema, you also need to learn how the increased stress of the pregnancy will affect your lymphedema. Your lymphedema therapist may be able to help you.

Communicating With People Outside Your Family

We have talked about dealing with the reactions of family and intimate partners. Now let's turn to more distant relationships.

Most people will know nothing about lymphedema. Think about how comfortable you are sharing information. What do you want to say, and to whom?

Lymphedema is not something to be ashamed of and some people find it empowering to educate others about the condition. You may find that sharing your knowledge makes you more comfortable and confident. It may put your listeners more at ease. As you speak openly about your condition, you may find that many other people have personal experience with chronic illness.

At the same time, you are under no obligation to answer a question just because it is asked. You have the right to refuse. You have the right to your privacy. You have the right to decide.

You don't have to use all the communication skills in more distant relationships. What you say to people and how much you share about your lymphedema depends on many factors. I'll explain three basic guidelines for dealing with other people.

As discussed in Chapter 10: Handling Others' Reactions, you may encounter some awkwardness or even prejudice from others. Friends, acquaintances, and/or coworkers may know you have lymphedema. If you work, your boss may have special concerns because you have a chronic medical problem. Your lymphedema may be visible to strangers.

We'll cover specific tips for dealing with each of these groups, and for dealing with healthcare providers.

Three Basic Communication Guidelines

You may find it helpful to follow these three communication guidelines in dealing with people with whom you do not share a close relationship. The guidelines are:

1. You get to decide what you say, how much you say, and to whom you say it.

2. You plan and practice what you choose to say.

3. You plan and practice how to say it, until you are as comfortable as possible.

Guideline 1: You Decide

Think about all the people you deal with in the course of daily life. They range from total strangers to close friends.

Worksheet 18-2: Focus on Pleasure

My Spontaneous Thoughts	Do They Increase or Decrease Pleasure?	Pleasurable Replacements (New Thoughts, Images, Etc.)

Among your acquaintances, neighbors, and coworkers, some are as distant as strangers, while other are as close as family. In fact, sometimes friends seem closer than family. You may share emotions more easily and they may be able to offer support and acceptance more easily because they are not so involved.

Think about which people know about your lymphedema or may notice physical changes from lymphedema. Usually visible differences make others nervous and when they are nervous they can be rude.

Remember, this may not be because they are rude people generally. It is often because they don't know what to do or how to react.

You are actually in a position of strength because you know what is going on. You can help them. You can choose your response to their reactions.

Guideline 2: Plan and Practice What to Say

Think about how others react. What reactions do you (or might you) encounter? What might other people say or do?

Now think about how you wish to handle these situations. What will you say and do? Decide exactly what information you wish to give.

(Dealing with bosses, managers, and supervisors is a special case. You will read about that a little later on and will decide at that point how you want to handle their reactions and concerns.)

Prepare a series of responses for strangers, acquaintances, friends, and coworkers. Your response may vary based on the specific person, the type of relationship you have with the person, and/or their specific reaction.

Plan ahead of time. Decide what you will say in different circumstances. Use worksheet 18-3 on page 301.

In completing the worksheet above, you decided on your responses and wrote them down. Your next step is to rehearse your responses.

Guideline 3: Plan and Practice How to Say It

You just completed planning the "what" of your response. Now you will plan and practice the "how."

Worksheet 18-3: My Planned Responses - Friends, Co-workers, Strangers

Type of Relationship	Other Person's Reaction, Statement, or Question	My Planned Response
Friend		
Acquaintance		
Coworker		
Strangers		

How you say something is as important as what you say. How you act with people affects how they act toward you.

Research shows that these factors make a positive difference:

- Make frequent eye contact

- Smile

- Nod often

- Speak using a calm, civil, mildly friendly tone of voice

- Stand and move comfortably and confidently

How we approach others strongly influences their reactions to us. When you behave this way, you help others interact better with you.

The more comfortable and at ease you are with yourself and with others, the more likely they are to be comfortable and at ease with you. People will be more likely to see you as a whole, unique, individual, as opposed to just seeing your lymphedema.

The web site www.changingfaces.org.uk has excellent tips for creating skillful and successful interactions with others. The web site was developed by and for people with facial deformities. It has many examples and stories of people who, despite being visibly different, are comfortable with others and deal skillfully with others' reactions.[3]

The more you practice speaking in a firmly civil and friendly voice while making eye contact, smiling and nodding to encourage the other person, the better your chance of feeling good and confident about dealing with others' reactions. Plus, the more practiced and confident you are, the more positive responses you are likely to elicit from others.

Practice your responses out loud. Continue practicing until you feel comfortable saying them.

Get feedback as you practice so that you improve. Practice until you have the skills "down cold," This helps you use the skills even if you're nervous or in a difficult situation.

Here are some suggestions on practicing:

- Practice the "how" skills in front of a mirror.

- Rehearse your planned responses using the skills on videotape. Review the video. Notice your increasing skill and comfort.

- Practice with a partner who will give you feedback.

- Rehearse and rehearse until you are comfortable with how you look and with what you say.

- Practice until you use the skills even when you feel self-conscious or nervous.

The most important tip is to go out and use the skills. Always remember Eleanor Roosevelt's words, *"No one can make you feel inferior without your consent."*[4]

Communicating with Coworkers

Your coworkers generally have two sets of concerns about you: personal and work-related. On a personal basis, they may worry about you and how lymphedema can affect your health. On a work-related basis, they are likely to worry about the effect of your condition on the organization.

There are some common concerns your coworkers may have. They may wonder:

- Are you liable to become ill at any time?

- Are you in pain?

- Are you going to die?

- Are you contagious? Will coworkers get lymphedema from you?

- Will you be able to do your job?

Check the boxes of the concerns you think your coworkers have. Write in any additional concerns now.

_____

_____

_____

Look at your answers to Worksheet 18-3: My Planned Responses on page 301. Are there more reactions or questions that you need to add in the Coworker section? If so, add them now.

Decide how to address these concerns. Choose ways that are acceptable to you. Don't ignore them. Write your planned response in the last column of the worksheet.

Communicating With Superiors at Work

Your bosses, managers, or supervisors are in a special situation. They decide whether to keep you on in your job, whether to promote you, and whether to fire you. For these reasons, you want to prepare your responses even more carefully.

Their Concerns

They may share some or all of your coworkers' personal and job-related concerns. They will have additional work-related questions.

Depending on the kind and size of the business they may worry about whether your condition will increase their cost of doing business. People with a visible difference tend to be seen as less competent. They may have more questions if they are thinking of promoting you.

Here are some likely concerns they may have:

- ☐ Can you do your job? What value do you bring to the company?

- ☐ Will they be caught short with your work undone?

- ☐ Will they need to hire more help?

- ☐ Will you need workplace accommodations? If so, how extensive will these be and how much will they cost?

- ☐ Will your condition increase the company's health insurance or worker's compensation insurance costs?

- ☐ If you have visible swelling or wear visible bandages or compression garments, will this create a negative image for the company?

- ☐ Is the company better off retaining you as an employee or firing you? Are there legal issues to be considered?

Check the boxes next to the concerns that you think your boss, manager, or supervisor have. Write these and any additional concerns that you have identified in the left column of Worksheet 18-4 on page 305.

Worksheet 18-4: My Planned Responses - Boss, Manager, or Supervisor

Reaction, Question, or Concern	My Planned Response	Communication Skills I Will Use

Your Responses

Decide how to address these concerns. Choose ways that are acceptable to you. Don't ignore them. Write your planned response in the second column of the worksheet on page 305.

Plan to use the communications skills mentioned above and note the skills you plan to use in the right hand column of the worksheet. Use tone of voice, eye contact, smiling, and nodding to decrease their discomfort and to show that you are comfortable, confident, and approachable.

Help your superiors express their concerns. Speak up for yourself as appropriate. Actively work with them to address their concerns in a way that is respectful and acceptable to both of you.

Because they have more power in the relationship, you need to work extra hard to make them feel that you understand and appreciate their concerns and are working with them.

The book, **Difficult Conversations**, has good work-related examples of using basic communication skills. You will find it under **Resources** at the end of this chapter.

By completing this worksheet, you decided on your responses and wrote them down. Your next step is to rehearse your responses.

Practice your responses out loud. Continue practicing until you feel comfortable and fluent saying them.

If You Think You Are Being Discriminated Against

If you think that you are being discriminated against because of your lymphedema, there are federal and state laws that may protect you. Federal laws that might apply include the Americans with Disabilities Act (ADA) and the Family and Medical Leave Act (FMLA).

You may want to start by asking yourself:

- Do I have actual evidence of discrimination?

- Does the evidence suggest that the discrimination is because of my lymphedema?

- How can I find out which federal or state laws apply to my situation?

- Who can give me information?

- Who can help me resolve this situation?

- What are my options? What are the pros and cons and the likely outcomes of each option?

You may want to talk with your human resources department, your union, or an attorney or mediator specializing in employment and disability law issues.

Communicating With Strangers

If your lymphedema is visible, strangers may respond positively or negatively. They may make offers of help. They may be eager to open doors or help with heavy lifting. They may express concern in a caring, respectful manner.

On the more negative side, strangers may either avoid making eye contact with you or they may stare. They may avoid talking to you or they may ask intrusive questions.

Always remember that while others do respond to our appearance, research has clearly shown that our manner and actions can counteract the effects of appearance. When others seem uncomfortable in your presence, they may be responding more to your actions than to your appearance.

The communication skills for dealing with strangers are similar to those for dealing with bosses, managers, and supervisors. These actions, which are listed here, are proven to powerfully impact others' reactions and impressions.

- Hold yourself in a relaxed, friendly, and confident manner.

- Use a firm, civil, confidently friendly tone of voice.

- Keep your head up.

- Deliberately make eye contact.

- Smile often.

- Nod frequently.

- Practice these actions until you do them skillfully.

Communicating with Healthcare Professionals

Communicating well with your healthcare team is important and can be difficult. This issue comes at the end of the chapter because, when talking with your healthcare team, you may use all the communication skills covered so far.

Protecting Yourself

Sometimes phlebotomists (lab technicians who draw blood for tests), medical assistants, paramedics, nurses, or other health professionals do not understand lymphedema precautions. They may try to draw blood, give injections, or take blood pressure using a limb with lymphedema.

See books like **Living Well with Lymphedema** and websites like www.LymphNotes.com and www.lymphnet.org for recommendations such as carrying a note from your physician or wearing a lymphedema alert bracelet on the limb.

You must speak up clearly and firmly to protect your health. You must act effectively even if it is uncomfortable.

Different Areas of Knowledge

Ideally, you should have a shared understanding with every healthcare professional that everyone is working together as a team. Each of you plays a vital role in ensuring the success of your partnership. Each of you has different expertise and carries different responsibilities.

My father, now retired, was a physician with a passionate commitment to the welfare of his patients and a tremendous awareness of the need for effective communication. He would say to his patients, *"You need to talk to me. I'm the mechanic, but you have the user's manual. You have to help me. This is your car I'm working on. It's you, your body. I can tell you what your options are, but you have to tell me what's going on and what you want."*[5]

You should expect that every professional you see has expert knowledge of some sort. Depending on the field and training, that might be expert knowledge about lymphedema, about the body as a whole, or about how various factors interact physiologically.

On your side of the team, you are the expert on you. Only you know what happens on a day-to-day basis. You have knowledge about your body, about its sensations and reactions, and about what actions you are currently taking. You know your emotions and your thoughts. You know your values, your concerns, and your questions.

Sharing Information about Lymphedema

Sometimes you have information about lymphedema that you wish to share with your healthcare provider. This can be a delicate issue. Here are some suggestions:

- Whenever possible, give them scientific evidence, rather than stories, conclusions, or assertions. Give them facts. Let them draw their own conclusions.

- Find reputable, credible sources of information.

- Professional peer-reviewed journals or the newsletters published by healthcare professional organizations are considered more reputable than general magazines or newspapers. Publications in the healthcare professional's own specialty may be viewed as more relevant or credible than publications from other specialties or from other fields.

- Websites displaying the HONcode logo are regarded as more reputable than websites without it. (This logo verifies that the website complies with the Health on the Net principles, www.hon.ch, designed to increase the accuracy, objectivity, and trustworthiness of health information offered on the Internet.)

- Chapter 24 of this book was written expressly for healthcare professionals and includes medical resources.

- Whenever possible, give them copies of written information so they can review or share the information if they wish.

- See the books under Talking to Healthcare Professionals in **Resources** at the end of this chapter.

- Use the communication skills. Practice ahead of time.

Ideally, any professional is eager to learn from anyone.

Questions and Answers

Any professional you see should be able to answer your questions so that you understand the answers. They should be able to explain the basis for their answers, whether it is logic, clinical experience, scientific research, accepted practice, or some combination of the four.

They should be able to explain things in words you understand. They should be able to explain the pros and cons, risks and benefits, the alternatives, and the likely outcomes. They should be honest with you about what they don't know and about the level of certainty or uncertainty in what they're telling you.

You need to figure out what questions you have. Having done that, you need to ask those questions.

You need to speak up when you don't understand something. Speak up when you disagree with what they say or are concerned or confused about their recommendations. Explain why you disagree or have concerns and be curious about the reasons and logic behind what they are saying.

Realistic Expectations

You have a right to expect certain things from your healthcare professionals. For example, you should expect them to:

☐ Treat you with respect.

☐ Be honest with you.

☐ Act ethically toward you.

☐ Keep current with the research and scientific advances in their field.

☐ Answer your questions.

☐ Work with you when suggesting treatment plans.

Check the boxes if these expectations are being met. If they are not being met, consider what steps you will take to improve things.

Your healthcare professionals have a right to expect certain things from you. For example, they should expect you to:

☐ Treat them with respect.

☐ Be honest when you report information or answer questions.

☐ Tell them about problems or changes.

☐ Ask questions, while recognizing that they don't have unlimited time.

☐ Do your best to carry out the treatment plan you have agreed to.

Check the boxes if you are meeting these expectations. If you are not doing your share, consider what steps you can take to improve things.

Unrealistic Expectations

Communication between you and your healthcare professionals can be complicated by unrealistic expectations on either side. Unrealistic expectations are common and contribute to mutual dissatisfaction and poor care.

Healthcare professionals may have unrealistic expectations of you and of themselves. They may expect that:

- You will never question them, their expertise, or their judgment.

- You will always agree with their conclusions, recommendations, views, and values regarding your condition and never want a second opinion.

- You will understand medical terminology exactly as they do.

- You will immediately comprehend information and instructions, even when it is new, complicated, and/or upsetting.

- You will not show emotions or have emotional reactions. If you do, they don't have to respond.

- You will remember everything without having it written down or repeated.

- If something doesn't work, it's your fault.

- They must (or do) know everything about everything.

- They have an answer for everything and are always be right.

You may share some of the unrealistic expectations listed **above. You** may also expect that:

☐ All the professionals you see will share your interpersonal **style and** you will like them personally.

☐ They will do what you want them to do.

☐ They will know what you want without your telling them.

☐ They will have an answer or a cure for everything. A particularly unrealistic expectation is that they will fix everything, without effort on your part.

☐ All professionals know about all areas of health. All professionals are equal regardless of field, training, experience, or knowledge.

☐ All web sites and sources of information are accurate, objective, and apply to you.

☐ You don't have to prepare for visits.

☐ You will never need to question or negotiate. Every treatment plan will be practical and acceptable to you.

☐ If something doesn't work, it's their fault.

Check off any of your unrealistic expectations that you recognize in this list. Think about how you can adjust your expectations and what you can do differently to get a more satisfactory outcome.

Emotional Matters

Care for lymphedema triggers all kinds of emotions. We have to undress for healthcare providers and be touched, poked, prodded, stretched, wrapped, measured, evaluated, and massaged. We have to deal with insurance coverage and paperwork in order to be reimbursed.

We may feel hope or despair, gratitude or anger, trust or mistrust, supported or abandoned, accepted or demeaned, proud or guilty and ashamed. Some of these emotions may stem from the past. Some may be simply a healthy emotional reaction to the situation. Some may be signals that you need to communicate with or change members of your treatment team.

Take a moment now to write down the feelings you have about your current healthcare team.

_____

_____

_____

Now, write down what you plan to do to lessen any negative emotions.

_____

_____

_____

Whenever you think your negative emotion is a result of a problem with your healthcare team, I encourage you to talk this over with them. Practice and use all the communication skills taught earlier in the chapter. If you can't resolve these feelings, consider whether you need to change health care providers.

If you have a repeated pattern of similar negative feelings or interactions with several healthcare providers despite differences among them, consider whether something from your past or in your present may be contributing to this unsatisfactory result. Reread any of the earlier chapters that are relevant. Apply some of the thinking and action skills from Chapters 16 and 17. Consider what you can do to get a more satisfying result.

Now add any additional ideas you have to your plan above.

Practical Matters

Sometimes communication falters because of simple, practical reasons. Here are suggestions that many people have found helpful:

- ☐ Before the visit, take time to identify your questions, concerns, and goals.

- ☐ Prioritize them and write them down, most important first, so the most important get covered first.

☐ Bring two copies of the list with you: one for you and one for the professional so both of you are, literally, "on the same page" in terms of what needs to be accomplished in the visit.

☐ Bring another person with you. Two memories are better than one. Plus, the other person may be able to better comprehend simply because they're less emotionally involved than you are.

☐ Plan a way to record the information. You can take notes, have someone else take notes, and/or (with permission) record the visit to review later.

☐ If everything that is on your list doesn't get covered in the visit, don't leave without a plan for when and how the remaining items will be addressed.

Check the ideas that you will try. Write down any other ideas you have.

_____

_____

_____

Sometimes You Have To Say Goodbye

Sometimes you can improve your communication and relationship with your healthcare provider. Sometimes you can't. You may feel dissatisfied despite your efforts to improve the situation. In this case, if you have the option to change caregivers, your most important communication skill may be to ask to see a different healthcare professional.

Resources

General Communication Skills

Difficult Conversations: How to Discuss What Matters Most by Douglas Stone, Bruce Patton, and Sheila Heen. Penguin Putnam, 1999.

Messages: The Communication Skills Book 2nd Edition by Matthew McKay, PhD, Martha Davis, PhD, and Patrick Fanning. New Harbinger Publications, 1995.

315 Chapter 18— Communication Skills   **315**

Assertiveness Skills

When I Say No, I Feel Guilty by Manuel Smith, PhD, Bantam Books, 1975.

Your Perfect Right: Assertiveness and Equality in Your Life and Relationships (8th Ed.) by Robert Alberti, PhD and Michael Emmons, PhD. Impact Publishers, 2001.

Couples Communication Skills

Fighting for Your Marriage: Positive Steps for Preventing Divorce and Preserving a Lasting Love by Howard Markman, PhD, Scott Stanley, PhD, and Susan Blumberg, PhD. Jossey-Bass, 1996.

Love is Never Enough: How Couples can Overcome Misunderstandings, Resolve Conflicts, and Solve Relationship Problems through Cognitive Therapy by Aaron Beck, MD. Harper Collins, 1989.

Passage to Intimacy by Lori Gordon, PhD and Jon Frandsen. Fireside, 2001.

The Relationship Cure: A 5 Step Guide to Strengthening Your Marriage, Family, and Friendships by John Gottman. Three Rivers Press, 2002.

The Seven Principles for Making Marriage Work by John Gottman and Nan Silver. Three Rivers Press, 2000.

We Can Work It Out by Clifford Notarius, PhD and Howard Markman, PhD. Putnam, 1993.

Why Marriages Succeed Or Fail: And How You Can Make Yours Last by John Gottman. Simon & Schuster, 1995.

Sexuality Issues

Becoming Orgasmic: A Sexual and Personal Growth Program for Women by Julie Heiman, PhD and Joseph LoPiccolo, PhD. Fireside, 1987.

For Each Other: Sharing Sexual Intimacy by Lonnie Barbach, PhD. Signet Books, 2001.

In Sickness and Health: Sex, Love, and Chronic Illness by Lucille Carlton. Delacorte Press, 1996.

The New Male Sexuality, Revised Edition by Bernie Zilbergeld, PhD. Bantam Books, 1999.

Talking With Children

Parenting Through Crisis: Helping Kids In Times Of Loss, Grief, And Change by Barbara Coloroso. Harper Collins, 2000.

How To Talk So Kids Will Listen And Listen So Kids Will Talk by Adele Faber and Elaine Mazlish. Avon Books, 1999.

Talking With Healthcare Professionals

The Intelligent Patient's Guide To The Doctor-Patient Relationship: Learning How To Talk So Your Doctor Will Listen by Barbara Korsch, MD and Caroline Harding. Oxford University Press, 1997.

Working With Your Doctor: Getting the Healthcare You Deserve by Nancy Keene. Patient Center Guides, 1998.

Notes

1   Why Marriages Succeed Or Fail: And How You Can Make Yours Last by John Gottman. Simon & Schuster, 1995.

2   According to some estimates, up to 45 percent of persons age 85 years and older have significant cognitive impairment and dementia. This information comes from www.apa.org/pi/aging/depression.html and is based on data from "The epidemiology of common late-life mental disorders in the community: Themes for the new century" by Gallo, J.J., & Lebowitz, B.D. (1999). *Psychiatric Services, 50*(9), 1158-1166.

3   www.changingfaces.org.uk

4   Familiar Quotations 14th Edition by John Bartlett, Ed. Emily Morison Beck. Boston: Little, Brown and Company, 1968.

5   Edmund B. McMahon, MD Private communication, June 23, 2005.

Chapter 19:
Professional Help

If, despite your best efforts, you aren't reaching your goals, consider seeing a mental health professional. You probably use experts for help with medical care, car repair, plumbing or electrical problems. Why not go to an expert for emotional problems? After all, you do deserve the best!

Only You Know What You Want

Before you see any professional, think about what you want to achieve. I cannot stress too much how important I believe this is.

It is comforting to talk to an accepting listener. It can be intellectually engaging to look back at your past. But talk by itself does not result in meaningful change. Sadly, it is possible to spend months or years in psychotherapy without making any significant change.

The bottom line is what do you really want? Are you making changes? Are you achieving your goals? How do you know?

Answer these questions as you start psychotherapy:

1. What is my goal? _____

2. What will be the early signs that I am making progress toward that goal? _____

3. What would be warning signs that therapy is not progressing? _____

4. How will I, and the professional I'm seeing, know when it is time to change or stop treatment? _____

What You Should Expect

You should feel respect and trust in any professional you see. What they say should make logical sense to you and should fit your experience. You should feel that they listen, understand, and treat you with respect.

At times, psychotherapy may be uncomfortable, difficult, or challenging. This is especially likely if you are dealing with fears, negative core beliefs, or past traumas. Generally, however, you should feel that you are in a mutually respectful, caring partnership.

Do Your Part

You are an active partner in treatment. Do your part. In many ways, what you do is more important than what the therapist does.

Talk with your therapist about questions or concerns that you have. Discuss conflicts and mixed feelings. You may wish to have your therapist read Chapter 25.

Review with your therapist your answers to the questions above. Both of you should understand what you want to achieve. Reach an agreement about the goals of treatment.

Work hard outside the session. Think about what was discussed in session. Experiment with new ideas or skills. Apply what you have learned.

If medication is prescribed, make sure you understand how to take it, what to expect, and what would be signs of problems. Call your healthcare provider if you have questions or problems. Then take the medicine as directed. Medicine can't work if you don't take it.

Locating Help

Your insurance company may have a list of qualified mental health professionals. Your physician, other healthcare professionals, friends, family members, or others with lymphedema may know licensed mental health professionals whom they recommend.

Many of the skills described in this section come from the cognitive-behavioral psychotherapy approach. If you are interested specifically in this approach, you may want to contact the National Association of Cognitive-Behavioral Therapists via their web site (www.nacbt.org) or by phone (1-800-853-1135).

You can also contact your state or local mental health association. Other sources of information and referrals are the national or state associations for psychiatrists, psychologists, social workers, marriage counselors, and psychiatric nurses.

Who Is A Licensed Mental Health Professional?

Licensed clinical psychologists or licensed psychiatric clinical social workers usually provide psychotherapy. Licensed registered nurses with specialty training in psychiatric nursing or licensed marriage counselors can also provide counseling or psychotherapy.

A psychiatrist is a licensed medical doctor who has received special training in treating emotional problems. This training is usually focused on using medication rather than psychotherapy, but this will vary from psychiatrist to psychiatrist.

Any licensed medical doctor can prescribe any medicine, including psychiatric medications. You don't have to see a psychiatrist to get medicines such as antidepressants. However, if you have the option, there can be benefits to having psychiatric medication prescribed by a specialist since psychiatrists may be more familiar with the latest medications and most effective dosages.

While licensure does not guarantee that a particular mental health professional will be effective, empathic, ethical, or right for you, it at least guarantees that the person has had recognized training and demonstrated a certain level of expert knowledge. If a licensed mental health professional behaves unethically or illegally, the state board that regulates their profession may be able to assist you.

Trainees

Students who are receiving professional training may offer counseling or psychotherapy under the supervision of a licensed therapist. There are some advantages to seeing a trainee, if you have that option. You may pay less per session and they may have more time to see you.

You should be told if you see a trainee and reassured that the trainee is being supervised and that your case will be discussed and overseen by the licensed supervisor. This is ethical. Similarly, in a medical center, you may see medical students or residents who are in training and who are being supervised by licensed physicians.

Unlicensed Therapists

Certain professional titles, like the ones just described above, are legally protected. By law, a person cannot use that title unless he or she has completed required training and passed required examinations established by state boards and has been licensed by the state.

Many other impressive-sounding titles are used but have no legal standing or licensure requirements. For example in most states, anyone can advertise that they are a "therapist," "counselor," "life coach," "healer," "neuro-linguistic programmer," "master certified hypnotherapist," "psychic," "trainer," and so on.

Training programs that bestow unlicensed titles can be offered without any research to demonstrate the effectiveness of the training or the therapy. Fancy diplomas can be printed and awarded stating that the person is "certified" in almost anything. However, being certified by an educational organization is *not* the same as licensed by the state. Unlicensed therapists generally do not rely on clinical research to find effective treatments.

This is a situation where *"Buyer Beware"* is good advice.

Protecting Positive Change

As you make positive changes, your challenge becomes maintaining your gains and accomplishments. This section includes ideas on:

- Supporting and maintaining positive changes.

- Avoiding burnout.

- Coping effectively.

- Monitoring how you are doing.

Chapter 20:
Maintaining Change and Preventing Burnout

Your final challenge is to support and maintain positive changes while preventing burnout. After all, caring for lymphedema is a lifelong task.

Give yourself time for the changes you are making to work. It has been said that it takes on average 12 months to adapt emotionally to the reality of a chronic illness. Each day brings you closer to feeling better if you use it to work toward your goals.

Accept that life is not static. Recall the saying, *"Life is a journey."* Neither your lymphedema nor your emotions will reach some perfect stable state.

Changes will occur in your life, your relationships, and your body. You may cycle through old, familiar emotional issues or confront new ones.

Your task, when this happens, is to respond effectively. Read whatever parts of this book are now relevant. Review chapters that helped before. Restart old skills or learn new ones.

Where Are You Now?

As you think about where you are now, what you have accomplished, and what comes next, three worksheets will be particularly helpful:

1. **Worksheet 14-2: My Emotional Challenges** (on page 201) was introduced in Chapter 1; by the end of Chapter 14 you had identified and prioritized the challenges facing you.

2. **Worksheet 14-3: How I Will Know I Have Reached My Goals** (on page 203) is where you defined personal goals and decided how you would measure progress.

3. **Worksheet 15-1: My Master Plan** (on page 225) is where you decided where you were in the process of change for your highest priority goals and chose the types of action needed.

Checking In

Blank copies of these three worksheets are included here so you can use them as thermometers to take your "emotional temperature" and get feedback on how you are doing. Make several copies of each to use to track your progress over the next several months.

In the first column, list your top priority goals. Get this information from Worksheet 14-3: How I Will Know I Have Reached My Goals.

In the second column, write down your best estimate of which step you are on right now in the change process for each goal. Then, in the third column, write the types of actions that match that step.

If you are confused about the second or third columns, review Chapter 15: The Five Steps of Change.

Where Are You Going?

I asked you to make several copies of each worksheet because you will use them over the next several months.

Make a note in your calendar to fill one out every month. Answer the questions without looking at your past answers. This gives you a snapshot of where you are. Then compare your current answers to your past answers to measure your progress.

If you have:

*   **Reached your goals:** Congratulations! Keep doing what you are doing. It is obviously working! Use actions from Step 5 in the stages of changes to maintain your gains.

Gloria's Story

I had two infections last year. The second one landed me in the hospital on IV antibiotics for a long time. I took a real honest look at my daily routine. My lymphedema therapist had told me what to do at home but I'd get busy and put it off. Well, I decided I couldn't put it off any longer. I really didn't want another infection.

I set several goals for myself. I learned the early signs of infection and check for them every day. My doctor and I decided what I should do if I think an infection is starting. And I really committed to daily self-care.

I bought a monthly calendar and hung it up. Every day, when I complete my self-management routine, I put a check mark in the box for that day. My sister gives me a CD each time I complete my self-management every day for a month. We go out to lunch to celebrate and she tells me how proud she is of me.

I haven't had an infection in months. The swelling's down. My doctor's pleased. So am I. Whenever I start to think that I'm doing so well I can skip my routine for the day, I look at that calendar with checkmarks in every box. I don't want any empty squares.

If I'm having a rough day, I call up my sister. She reminds me of how bad I felt in the hospital and how good I feel now and I remember why I need to do it every day.

I feel so much better and not just physically, either. I don't worry and feel scared like I did before. I'm proud of how much better I look. I go out and do more. Life is good and I plan to keep it that way.

- **Not yet reached your goal but see steady progress:** Continue whatever you are doing that is making progress possible. You can also try additional techniques, reread relevant parts of this book, and/or seek more help.

- **Lost gains you had made, or your progress has stalled and you are dissatisfied with where you are:** Examine what you are doing (or not doing). Are you using the skills in the book? Where are you in the stages of change? Do you need to restart what you did in the past that led to progress? Do you need to use different techniques?

- **Maintained your gains but face new challenges:** Turn to the relevant chapters and tackle the current challenges. Sometimes having a new challenge appear in our lives is actually a sign of progress. For example, having to deal with others' reactions and learn new communication skills is a sign of progress if, in the past, you were so overwhelmed or self-conscious that you basically had no relationships with others.

What Can You Expect?

There are predictable challenges in maintaining a positive change over time. Let's look at some of the rough spots you can expect and how to get over them.

Enjoy those times when things go smoothly. Don't be shocked or discouraged when difficulties arise. Expect to experience some emotional flare-ups. Your body is not static. Your emotions are not static. Life is not static.

Boredom

The initial excitement of tackling or overcoming a challenge will wane. In general, whenever we do something regularly, our emotional reaction to it tends to lessen.

In some situations, this decrease in emotion is positive. For example, fear of making a mistake in self-care lessens with practice. Or if you are anxious about advocating for yourself, you will feel more comfortable, the more you speak up. When you face your fears regularly, deliberately and effectively, you become less afraid.

However, there are situations when having lessened emotional reactions is a problem. For example, it can be very exciting when you first see positive results from lymphedema treatment. But the novelty wears off, the excitement lessens, and boredom sets in.

Or maybe you use the skills in this book to lift your mood or improve your communication. But then the excitement of using new skills and seeing results diminishes; you find yourself not wanting to make the effort.

How will you maintain your daily regimen year after year? What will motivate you? Relying solely on emotional responses, such as fear or excitement, to provide your motivation is a weak strategy.

Worksheet 20-1: My Emotional Challenges

Emotional Challenge	Severity Rating 0 – 10	Coping Rating 0 - 10	Red Flag? Y/N	My Priorities
Feeling overwhelmed				
Sadness and grieving				
Anger and resentment				
Fear				
Self-protection				
Worry				
Increased body focus				
Self-consciousness				
Others' reactions				
Searching for meaning				
Trauma and core beliefs				
Current stress				

Pam's Story

Soon after my breast cancer treatment, I was diagnosed with lymphedema. I consider myself fortunate because my physician diagnosed it promptly and referred me to an excellent treatment facility. My mindset was, "*I beat the cancer. I can manage this too.*"

That was five years ago. I have learned to manage and live with lymphedema. However, there are times when I "*hit the wall*" emotionally.

During these dark times, I really hate having lymphedema. I hate the swelling; hate the treatment regimen. I long for time out. Just one day, well maybe more than one, without being aware of the lymphedema and particularly without wearing that ugly sleeve.

I have learned to help myself get through these times by thinking about my friend, Giselle, who is diabetic. I think about how diabetics don't get a day off. In fact I know that Giselle doesn't even get an hour off from monitoring her blood sugar, measuring what she eats, and balancing this with how much she exercises. Thinking about Giselle helps me keep going.

Don't assume you will stay excited. Assume you will get bored—and plan how you will continue your efforts despite that.

Coping Suggestions:

Expect the decrease in excitement.

Plan for boredom.

Think about what will keep you going even when you are bored.

Use Step Five ideas from Chapter 15: The Five Steps of Change.

Use ideas from Chapter 16: Thinking Skills.

Use ideas from Chapter 17: Action Skills.

Worksheet 20-2: How I Will Know I Have Reached My Goals

My Priority List of Challenges	My Goal For Severity Rating	My Goal For Coping Rating	Ways I Will Know I Have Reached My Goal

Lapses

You'd think that after going to all the trouble of deliberately making a successful and positive change that you would automatically stay changed. But, that is not the case.

We human beings have a natural tendency to fall back into old habits. We forget. We postpone. We procrastinate.

You can suddenly find yourself acting and reacting like you did in the past. This is natural and predictable. It is one of the reasons there is a maintenance step in the change process and it is one of the reasons this chapter was written.

66

I am good at bandaging at night for a while—and then I don't. **99**

Coping Suggestions:

Don't panic.

Don't get angry at yourself.

Don't give up.

Remind yourself lapses are natural.

Go back to Chapter 15. Figure out what step you are on *now* in the process of change for this issue. Once you know your step, restart actions for that step that worked for you in the past.

Repeat as needed until you are back in the maintenance stage.

Competing Demands

Expect that competing demands for your time, energy, and attention will tempt you to return to an old pattern of reacting or to turn your attention away from change. We all have legitimate demands that compete for our time or attention. Plus, modern life makes tempting distractions readily available. And old habits, whether of action of thinking or of feeling, occur more readily when we are tired or distracted.

Worksheet 20-3: My Master Plan

My Top Priority Goals	I'm At Step:___	Actions For This Step

> ### *Coping Suggestions:*
>
> Prepare for this reality. You can't do everything.
>
> Consider how you will choose and prioritize.
>
> Make a reasonable, doable, realistic priority list. Remember, you can't do everything.
>
> To sustain motivation, list every single reason, big and small, for working to feel better.
>
> Think about your long-term goals. Look at the big picture.

Crises

Apart from the demands of daily life, you will face crises in your life at times. Our emotions run higher during crises. Old habits are more likely to return when we are stressed.

> ### *Coping Suggestions:*
>
> Reflect on how you tend to react during crises.
>
> First, review what you have learned about emotional challenges and about yourself.
>
> Then, use this knowledge to plan how you will maintain good mental and physical self-care during stressful times.
>
> Decide how you will deal with emotional challenges if they temporarily resurface in response to a crisis.

What Can You Do?

Not surprisingly, some of the suggestions in this chapter come from the section in Chapter 15: The Five Steps of Change on Maintenance, Step Five in the change process.

Go back and quickly review your answers to the questions in that section or write answers now if you did not before. Add anything new that occurs to you now.

Take Maintenance Step Actions

Five actions that are helpful during the maintenance stage of change are:

1. Use praise and reward yourself for maintaining your changes.

2. Talk to others and teach them how to make and maintain changes.

3. Continue to track how you are doing.

4. Respond to early warning signals and restart change if you falter.

5. Recycle through the steps of change as needed.

Surround Yourself with Support

Find sources of continuing support that will last over the long haul. It can be easier to get support during a crisis or during the action stage of change. But support that continues over time helps you maintain changes. It also helps minimize feeling of being alone or abandoned.

Get support from your family, friends, lymphedema therapist, healthcare providers, support group, neighbors, religious group, online contacts, and any other source you can find. You are looking for people who will support you in continuing to overcome emotional challenges. Remember and review their helpful or encouraging comments.

Seek support from inspirational or motivating quotations, especially those that emphasize perseverance. Seek out inspiring examples of success and persistence.

Gain support from what you say as you praise and reward yourself. Gain support from stories of others who have overcome and maintained.

Speak Up

Ask for what you want. Let other people know when and how you would like them to support you in the changes you've made.

Tell people how you feel. Use the communication skills from Chapter 18 to negotiate for what you want or to improve your relationships.

One research study showed that people with chronic conditions who were more specific and assertive with their healthcare professionals had better results.[1] Reread Chapter 18: Communication Skills as often as you need.

Make It a Habit

Notice what you are doing to overcome your emotional challenges. Now, make it a habit—whether it is changing your thinking, changing your actions, or using your communication skills. Making something a habit is one of the best ways to maintain it over the long run.

Find ways to make your change actions become a "thoughtless" habit. In other words, create ways to make it part of your daily routine so that you do whatever you need to do, almost without thinking about it—as a matter of course.

Make It Easy

Make it easy to do. Get everything you may need in a convenient place. Minimize the number of steps, mental or physical.

For example, you might keep your tape, lotion, bandages, and foam together, organized, and next to where you use them. If you measure swelling on a chart, keep the tape and the chart together and easy to reach. If you are using a journal, chart, or worksheet to track progress on one of your challenges, keep it where it is handy to use.

Make it easy to remember. Build your changes into your daily routine. Make maintaining your changes as automatic as possible.

For example, have a regular time in your schedule for exercise or self-massage. Schedule time for doing one or more of the thinking or action skills, such as daily worry time, write-and-destroy writing, getting together with people, and so on.

Make It Non-Negotiable

Make maintaining your changes non-negotiable. As they say in labor-management negotiations, *"Take it off the table."*

Don't debate about maintaining your change. Don't discuss that option with yourself. Don't discuss it with other people. Don't let other people discuss it with you.

Treat maintaining your changes as a closed issue. This is not something that is open to being re-debated, re-negotiated, or re-decided. It is not a question where the answer varies with your mood at the moment.

You have made your changes. You have made your decision. You have made your commitment to health. This issue is decided. It is not open for renegotiation. Do what keeps you emotionally and physically healthy.

Build on Success

Record your successes. Keep a journal (or some other record) of your achievements, accomplishments, successes, and learnings. Focus on every instance of success, large or small.

Pay attention to what you do that makes those successes possible. Remember what works. Deliberately do more of what works.

Respond Quickly to Lapses

Remember, change is a process. At times, you are likely to lapse back into an earlier stage in the change process and again have difficulty with an emotional challenge.

Here is a possible scenario. Notice the changes in thoughts, feelings, and actions.

> Sue had succeeded in becoming more hopeful and beginning to actively take care of her lymphedema. Infections stopped and she was thrilled. Then her limb got infected.
>
> Even though the infection quickly responded to antibiotics, she now found herself thinking, *"My infections will never really improve. Why bother? This is hopeless. I ought to maintain my regimen but I don't want to."* She felt anxious, angry, hopeless, and guilty. She sought comfort by eating bags of chips while channel-surfing with the television remote. Meanwhile, she cancelled her therapist appointment and stopped self-massage and compression.

What are likely to be *your* warning signals that you are having a lapse?

_____

What old thoughts are likely to return?

_____

What old emotions are likely? Do you have specific challenges that tend to return?

What do you tend to do during a lapse?

If you notice any of these signs, reread the information and coping suggestions about lapses starting on page 330.

Deal with Other Problems if They Arise

Other emotional challenges can rear their ugly heads and start to undermine your progress. If this happens:

- Read the chapter(s) for the challenge(s) confronting you.

- Identify the coping suggestions you think will be most useful and follow those suggestions.

- If that's not enough, review Chapters 16-18 on All-Purpose Skills.

Notes

1   "Assessing the effects of physician-patient interactions on the outcomes of chronic disease." Kaplan SH, Greenfield S, Ware JE. *Med Care.* 1989; 27 (suppl 3) S110-S127.

Chapter 21

Good Coping and Ineffective Coping

If you have lymphedema, this is the final chapter written specifically for you. It is a summary chapter. This chapter reviews the essential lessons of this book, presents nine signs of good coping, and ends with six warning signs of poor coping.

What You Have Gained

By now you have learned a great deal. Think about the ideas, information, and awareness you have gained. Consider the knowledge and resources you have acquired.

At this point, you:

- Recognize the challenges you have successfully handled (congratulations!)
- Have identified any remaining challenges, set your goals, and can track progress
- Know the steps of change and what to do at each step
- Have powerful tools for change
- Know where to find more information

The Take Home Lessons

Here is a quick summary of key ideas I want you to take with you:

- Lymphedema presents emotional challenges that impact you and your life.

- You *can't* escape the emotional challenges. You *can* choose your response to them.

- You can respond actively and skillfully—or passively and poorly. You can choose to persist or to give up. You can choose to confront emotionally difficult areas and to learn, practice new skills, and grow—or you can choose to avoid.

- Your choices will affect you, physically and emotionally.

Nine Signs of Good Coping

Here is my nine-point summary of the signs of good coping.

1) Actively Taking Charge

People who carry out self-treatment of lymphedema have much better results. People who take an active approach to overcoming challenges tend to be happier, more confident, more successful, and find more people to help and support them.

If you are actively taking charge, you don't wait for others to see your needs and rescue you. You don't stew in anger, regret, or blame. You don't run and hide.

You tackle your challenges. You work toward your goals.

2) Educating Yourself

You identify and prioritize your problems. Then you get the information you need to solve or cope with them.

You ask your healthcare professionals. If they don't or can't answer your questions, you ask again or you ask others. You find people who are successful in solving these problems and ask them.

You learn from others' successes and failures. You read about lymphedema and about dealing with difficult emotions. You contact reputable websites. You join appropriate organizations.

3) Finding Solutions

You seek out treatment options. If needed, you change treatment providers. If one approach doesn't work, you find another. You keep looking until you discover what works best for you.

You actively seek treatment options and evaluate them. When treatments or specific actions are suggested, you evaluate them against your experience, the experience of others, scientific evidence, and logic.

You ask questions. You find answers. You communicate. You educate. You negotiate.

4) Recording What Works

You notice positive changes, however small or fleeting at first. You keep track of changes. You look for patterns and triggers.

You zero in on what makes things better. You pay attention to those times when your mood is better or your lymphedema improves. You ask yourself what are you doing differently that makes those improvements possible. Then you deliberately do more of that.

5) Educating and Helping Others

You share what you learn with your family and friends, with your healthcare professionals, and with others who have lymphedema. You may start or join a support group. You may participate in a chat room or online bulletin board.

Explaining to others what works is a good way to make it clearer in your own mind.

6) Finding Alternatives

As part of actively participating in treating your lymphedema, you create alternative ways of doing tasks – ways that protect your body or that help treat your lymphedema. You take lymphedema into account as you develop ways to do chores, enjoy pleasures, and engage in activities.

You learn what fosters mental and physical health and you act on that knowledge. You find new ways to cook, sew, garden, carry, lift, and clean. You problem-solve. You discover ways to exercise that help your lymph flow.

When possible, you adapt pleasurable activities so you can do them despite lymphedema. When activities you enjoyed are absolutely contraindicated because of lymphedema, you actively search out new pleasures.

You act on the saying "For every door that closes, another door opens." When you hit an obstacle, you set out to find a way over, under, around, or through it.

You fill your life with positives. You focus on solutions.

7) Facing Your Fears

You have learned that running and hiding out of fear simply guarantees that you stay afraid. Fear feeds fear. Trying to run from frightening thoughts makes them return more often and stronger.

We are coping beings. Look at the history of the human race. We would never have survived if we were not able to cope.

Whatever you fear, you recognize that you will be better off facing it head on. You remind yourself that, nearly all the time, fear is lying to you when it tells you that you can't cope and that fear presents dangers as much worse or more likely to happen than they really are.

You give yourself full credit for the things you have already coped with in your life. You reflect on times you faced problems head on and overcame them compared to times you ran from them and gave up.

You think about which approach worked better in the long run. You notice which approach made you feel better about yourself.

You act on that knowledge. You minimize acting out of fear. You support and encourage yourself. You applaud yourself for your courage in facing difficulties.

8) Treating Setbacks as Opportunities for Growth

You recognize that, while setbacks can be uncomfortable, embarrassing, frustrating, or inconvenient, they are chances to learn and grow. They are opportunities.

The truth is that we grow more through challenges and difficult times than we do through easy or comfortable times. It may not seem fair, but there it is.

A phrase that captures this essential concept is "Every problem comes bearing a gift in its hands." You tackle the problem in order to get the gift.

9) Finding Inspiring Examples of Success

You find role models. You focus on, recall, and repeat the encouraging words of others.

You deliberately cultivate a view of life that inspires and supports you. You fill your mind with examples of courage, acceptance, and perseverance like these mentioned below.

Mark Goldstein developed lymphedema after treatment for breast cancer. He has gone on to become a lymphedema advocate and a marathon runner. He emphasizes repeatedly that *"I realized [lymphedema] was giving me an opportunity....There are choices out there and we are empowered to make those choices. Make a decision. Choose a path."*[1]

Gary Hall, Jr., the swimmer, competed in three Olympics and won multiple gold medals despite having Type 1 diabetes. For him, having this chronic illness gave him *"...a sense of appreciation for who I am and what I am doing, and making every day count."*[2]

Helen Keller, who was both blind and deaf from childhood on, wrote, *"Although the world is full of suffering, it is full also of the overcoming of it."*[3]

If the Nine Signs of Good Coping Reflect How You Cope

If the signs of good coping sound familiar to you and reflect your actions, you are on a good path. By following these coping guidelines, you have an excellent chance of overcoming not only the challenges of lymphedema, but also any other challenges life may hand you.

Six Warning Signs of Ineffective Coping

Ineffective coping is marked by avoidance and passivity. Maybe you avoid responsibility by blaming others. Maybe you're spending your energy on anger rather than changing what you can.

Maybe you avoid persevering when things get hard, scary, boring, or discouraging. Maybe you avoid trying at all. Some research studies have found that passive, avoidant coping is associated with *more* emotional distress and *worse* lymphedema outcome.[4]

Here are six major signals of ineffective coping.

1) You Wait to be Rescued

Being rescued is a powerful fantasy. Think about how often it shows up in fairy tales, books, TV shows, and movies.

If you had a nurturing childhood, you may want to return to that blissful state. You were cared for without any work on your part.

If you didn't have such a childhood, you may have an even deeper yearning to experience what it would be like. In real adult life however, we rarely, if ever, get to be treated like this. We have to get to work and "rescue" ourselves.

If you are waiting for others to rescue you, have you noticed that it usually doesn't happen? When it doesn't happen, how do you feel?

You are likely to be stuck feeling angry, resentful, betrayed, sad, let down, helpless, or abandoned. Ask yourself if the emotional price you pay is worth clinging to a fantasy.

2) You Ask No Questions

Maybe in school or while growing up at home you were trained to not ask questions Maybe you still hesitate to ask questions. Maybe you don't want to upset anyone or challenge anyone or "make waves" or "make them upset or angry." You are still acting as if you were a child and as if you were still dealing with the same people. .

Things have changed. You are not a child any more. You are an adult with a chronic condition that you have to manage. You need to speak up and ask until you get the information you need.

Why? Because your body needs you and you are the only expert on your body and your emotions.

Only you know what questions you have. Only you know what information you need. Only you know when you do and don't understand something enough to use the information.

Your health care providers, family members, friends, and coworkers may all be knowledgeable and caring people, but they are not mind readers and never will be. If you don't ask, you won't know.

3) You Accept What Is Offered, Even if It Is Not What You Need

It is true that compromise and accepting what you can't change are essential life skills. But advocating and negotiating for what you need are equally essential skills.

It can be easy to just accept whatever is offered. The limitation with this approach is that no one knows what you need better than you do.

You need to protect and develop your mental and physical health.

You are not your healthcare professional's only patient or client. You are not the top priority to your insurance provider. You are not the only employee in your employer's business. You are the person primarily responsible for your health.

Remember, your body and your mind depend upon *you* to protect them. They can't step out and get what they need. They are entirely dependent on you.

Do you automatically settle for whatever is offered, regardless of the circumstances? Why do you accept whatever is offered and let it go at that?

Ask yourself:

• What am I telling myself?

_____

• How well is this strategy working?

_____

• If I do not take care of myself, who will?

_____

4) You Give Up All Activities

When you give up *all* activities, you don't decide and discover for yourself what changes you need to make and what changes you don't need to make. You don't monitor the effects of different activities on your lymphedema and your emotions. You don't prioritize. You don't problem-solve. You just give up everything.

Activity is important for many reasons. Muscle movements help move lymph and reduce lymphedema. Activities lift mood and self-esteem. They can give life meaning and can connect you to others.

Physically, the less you move, the less your muscles move the lymph. Emotionally, the fewer activities you are involved in, the narrower your world becomes. Inactivity and withdrawal make you weaker, sicker, and unhappier.

If you are caught in this pattern, ask yourself:

• Am I happy with this in the long run?

_____

• How does it make me feel physically and emotionally?

_____

• What are the costs?

_____

5) You Avoid or Hide From Other People

You may go to great efforts to hide your lymphedema from others. You may tell yourself that it is easier to hide than have to handle questions or stares.

It may seem easier, but consider what it takes away from you:

- You lose the opportunity to educate others.
- You lose the opportunity to accept yourself and your body.
- You lose the opportunity to learn which people will truly accept you.
- You lose the opportunity to diminish your fears.
- You lose chances for spontaneity and freedom.
- You let your fears keep you imprisoned.
- You lose the opportunity to increase confidence, self-respect, and acceptance.

Ask yourself whether hiding and avoiding are truly worth the hidden costs.

6) You Give Up and Blame Others or Life

You may have decided that you can't change. Because you can't change some things, you may have decided that it is not worth trying to change anything.

You may have concluded that change is useless or impossible. Maybe you tried more active coping and encountered setbacks. This happens.

It is painful and discouraging. It is unfortunate and unpleasant. It is a fact of life.

Think about this. Which is better: having to drive on a difficult, rough road in order to reach your destination or having no road to drive on at all?

Life is often a difficult road but when you give up, it is as though you turn off the car engine. You stop all chance of forward progress. You change a rough road into no road at all.

By all means, let yourself be upset when you hit an obstacle. Let yourself have a good cry about it if you like. Have a good temper tantrum about it. Feel your emotions. Let them out in safe ways. Do that as long and as often as you need.

Then pick yourself up, brush yourself off, step back to look at the whole situation, and figure out your next move. As Jesse Jackson once said, *"You are not responsible for being down, but you are responsible for getting up."*[5]

If the Six Warning Signs Reflect How You Cope

If any of the above six warning signs are familiar, you are almost certainly using ineffective strategies. These approaches interfere with overcoming your emotional challenges.

Praise yourself for noticing this. You may have a great deal to gain and noticing problems opens the door.

Now, it is probably time to take a different approach. If you:

- **Believe that specific emotional challenges are stopping you from coping more actively and effectively,** reread the chapters devoted to the relevant challenges.

- **Aren't ready to change at this time,** reread Chapters 14 and 15 on how to clarify your priorities, determine where you are in the process of change, and identify types of actions that you are ready to take and that would feel appropriate to you.

- **Are ready to change now,** reread Chapters 16-18: Tools for Change. Select specific skills from the toolkit. Apply them. Use worksheets to prioritize and track your progress.

- **Haven't succeeded on your own,** seek out support and help. If you are considering seeking professional help, reread Chapter 19.

Farewell and Good Luck

Regardless of how well or how poorly you are coping at this moment in time, I think you should be proud of yourself for reading this book. Doing that took time and effort. Thank you for reading.

You have exposed yourself to new ideas. You may have planted the seeds for future change.

We all have potential for change and growth, for joy and achievement. I hope with all my heart that you tap into your potential, more and more frequently. I hope you find this book helpful in that process.

May you reap the benefits of your efforts. May you live and be well. Take good care of yourself.

Notes

1   "We Are Hear!" keynote address by Mark A. Goldstein at the 2005 National Lymphedema Network International Patient Summit, Reno, NV on August 19, 2005.

2   "Gary Hall, Jr. An Olympian for the Third Time" by Daniel Trecroci. *Diabetes Health*, September, 2004.

3   **Seeking Safety: A Treatment Manual for PTSD and Substance Abuse** by Lisa Najavits. Guilford Press, 2001. (p. 100)

4   "Psychosocial aspects of upper extremity lymphedema in women treated for breast carcinoma" by S. Passik and M. McDonald. *Cancer* Supplement December 15, 1998; 83(12):28172820.
"Lymphedema: Strategies for management" by S. R. Cohen, D. K. Payne, and R. S. Tunkel. *Cancer*, Supplement August 15, 2001; 92(4):980-987.
"Predictors of psychological distress, sexual dysfunction and physical functioning among women with upper extremity lymphedema related to breast cancer" by S. D. Passik, et al. *Psychooncology* 1995; 4:255-263.

5   **Seeking Safety: A Treatment Manual for PTSD and Substance Abuse** by Lisa Najavits. Guilford Press, 2001. (p. 117)

Helping People
With Lymphedema

This section provides information for those who care for and care about people with lymphedema. Specific information is included for:

- Family and friends of people with lymphedema, Chapter 22.

- Parents of children with lymphedema, Chapter 23.

- Healthcare professionals of all types, Chapter 24.

- Mental health professionals, Chapter 25.

Chapter 22

For Family and Friends

If you have a family member or friend with lymphedema, this chapter was written for you. It covers common problems you may encounter and offers specific suggestions and additional resources.

If you read only this chapter, you will gain some useful skills. At the same time, I hope you will be interested enough to read the earlier chapters.

By reading more, you will gain a deeper understanding of lymphedema and of the emotional challenges your loved one is facing. That knowledge can strengthen your relationship. Plus, the ideas and skills throughout this book are useful in many areas of life.

Lymphedema Affects You as Well

66   *My husband has lymphedema in both legs that requires daily bandaging. He can't manage this by himself. Some days I feel as if I do nothing but take bandages off, wash bandages, roll bandages, and put bandages on. In between, I have to cook, clean, and drive the children to their activities and pick up the slack by taking on the jobs he can't do any more.*

I am so grateful that he is alive and basically healthy. But still, sometimes I feel trapped, you know, like I don't have a life of my own anymore **99**

The bad news is that when you have a close friend or family member with a chronic illness, it can affect you and it can stress your relationship. The good news is that relationships that survive become deeper and stronger.[1]

❝ The marriage vows…take on a whole new meaning….Here is a man who…would take me with or without breasts, with or without hair and eyebrows, and with an arm and hand that could look like a pincushion at any instant.[2] ❞

You care enough to be reading this chapter. That fact alone says a lot about your commitment to your partner and to the relationship.

Here are some common issues that family or friends encounter. Check the ones that apply to you:

☐ *"I want to help but don't know how. What can I do? How can I help with either the physical or the emotional demands of lymphedema?"*

☐ *"I feel sad seeing her struggle with lymphedema. I worry about her. I'm scared for her."*

☐ *"I feel guilty that I'm healthy."*

☐ *"I get impatient. I resent the demands lymphedema places on our lives."*

☐ *"I'm angry about how he handles his lymphedema."*

☐ *"We disagree about lymphedema management. Sometimes she asks me to do something I don't want to do."*

☐ *"How can I handle our disagreements and still protect our relationship?"*

List any other issues that you are facing.

_____

Lymphedema Related Issues Worksheet

Think about the issues that you and your loved one face and write them in the first column of worksheet 22-1 on page 353.

Next, ask yourself these questions:

1. What am I doing to resolve or cope with each issue? Write your answers in the second column of the worksheet.

2. How satisfied am I with the results of my current approach on a scale of 0 to 10? Write your answers in the third column of the worksheet.

3. What would I like to be different? Write your answers in the fourth column of the worksheet.

Worksheet 22-1: Lymphedema Related Issues

Issue	My Current Approach	How Satisfied?	What I Would Like To Be Different?

Writing things down is very helpful in dealing with problems. It forces you to use more of your brain. It slows down your thinking so you have a chance to be clearer, more detailed, and more logical. It gives you the opportunity to return and review what you have written.

The general skills in this chapter may be enough by themselves to resolve many problems, but some issues or emotions can be particularly upsetting or difficult. For issues that trigger a lot of emotion, read the earlier chapters about the specific emotions involved. Also, Chapters 16-18: **Tools for Change** will give you additional ideas and skills.

How Can I Help Them?

You are reading this chapter because you want to help. Here are five general suggestions that apply to basically any issue.

First: Listen For the Feelings

First of all, listen for the feelings behind the other person's words. This, by itself, may be one of the hardest and most important things you can do. Living with lymphedema is demanding. You want to be there for the other person.

Accept and acknowledge all their feelings, even the negative feelings. Empathize with the difficulties and problems. Accept the negative reactions. The person you care about will probably experience an entire range of emotions over time.

Dealing with lymphedema can be time-consuming, uncomfortable, frustrating, discouraging, and infuriating. At different times, or even simultaneously, someone with lymphedema may feel sad, hopeful, ashamed, fearful, excited, discouraged, proud, worried, grateful, and/or resentful.

Listen and accept whatever feelings they have at the time. This allows the other person to be truly heard, accepted, and understood.

Listening with acceptance and understanding gives the other person a chance to identify what's going on inside them. It offers the opportunity for you both to become closer to one another.

Sometimes just the act of putting thoughts and feelings into words helps people. More often than you might imagine, we don't really know what we think and feel until we start talking or writing and have to express our thoughts and feelings in words.

Avoid the Common Listening Mistakes

We frequently make two mistakes when we listen. Both mistakes stem from a desire to help and connect with the other person, yet both mistakes undermine our efforts. They are examples of good intentions resulting in ineffective actions. By knowing about these mistakes, you will be more able to avoid them.

The first common mistake is to immediately start solving problems. We want to help. We want the other person to feel better. We want them to avoid mistakes.

When we jump in with advice before completing the listening phase it is as if we jump to planting seeds in a garden without preparing the soil or starting to build a house without laying the foundation. Making sure the other person feels listened to and understood is the preparation and foundation necessary for having them become ready, in turn, to listen to us. If you want to be listened to, listen first.

The second common mistake is to jump in with our own feelings, thoughts, and stories. Again, this is an understandable mistake that stems from a laudable goal. We are searching our own experiences to find ways to connect with what others tell us.

Sometimes our reactions are very similar to those of the person who is talking and the speaker feels understood. Sometimes, however, we shift before the other person has had enough time to finish fully expressing their emotions and they feel cut off. Or, because each of us is different, our reactions are different from those of our friend or loved one.

Experiment with putting your own reactions, experiences, concerns, or criticisms on hold at first. Listen. Explore. Seek to understand things from their viewpoint.

Think how rare it is to have someone who really wants to know what you think and feel, who wants to know you as you are. Every time you can offer this to your friend or family member, you offer them a precious gift.

Second: Find the Positives

Deliberately find the positives in the person or in their actions. Even when they are not coping well with their lymphedema or their emotions, there are always positives somewhere. Your job is to notice them.

To help identify the positives, ask yourself these questions:

•   In what ways are they showing courage and actively coping?

   _____

•   Are they successfully managing their lymphedema problems and emotions at least some of the time? What are they doing during those times?

   _____

•   Are they doing self-management and acting to minimize flare-ups?

   _____

•   Are they aware of problems, even if they haven't found a good solution yet?

   _____

•   Are they being honest with you, even if they are not coping successfully?

   _____

•   What do you admire, love, appreciate, or respect about them?

   _____

•   What are their strengths and potentials?

   _____

Find those positives and acknowledge them in words. Help the other person see them. Tell them the potential you see in them. Share the hopes you have for them in the future.

Third: Encourage Active Coping

We can cope with physical and emotional challenges either passively or actively.

- Passive coping involves waiting for time to heal, waiting for others to fix problems, giving up, and/or refusing to take responsibility for coping.

- Active coping involves doing what needs to be done and what is possible, as well as actively seeking help from others.

Encourage the person you care about to cope actively with their lymphedema and to cope actively with their emotional reactions.

Research suggests that generally people with lymphedema who take an active approach to coping do better both physically and emotionally. Taking an active, rather than a passive, approach minimized lymphedema symptoms and improved the quality of life.[3]

Active coping is powerful. It is a person's best hope for doing well physically, coping well emotionally, and dealing well with others.

Fourth: Use Praise and Support

Look for all the ways in which the person *is* actively coping. Identify each action they have taken, even if those actions seem small or have not yet been successful. Be generous with your praise. Reward their positive efforts.

Be a cheerleader and support person for the other person. Keep telling them why and how you believe that they can cope well.

With words and actions, let your friend or loved one know that you care. Show them that you are there for them. Demonstrate your caring and support in ways that are meaningful to them.

Decades of research on behavior change, on influence, and on communication agree that positive approaches, like the ones you have been reading about above, result in more sustained change than negative approaches such as criticism, sarcasm, or punishment.

In general, when negative approaches are used, even if change occurs, the change tends to be short-lived and to come with certain predictable disadvantages and costs:

- After a period of time, the person usually goes back to the problem behavior that was criticized or punished.

- After returning to the old behavior the person will be more likely to hide the problem behavior or lie about it and less likely to admit or talk about the problem.

- Negative approaches usually create negative feelings such as shame, embarrassment, sadness, or anger.

- As a result of the above, the relationship between the people involved tends to worsen. There is more defensiveness, denial, or anger. There is less closeness, less honesty, and less trust.

There is certainly a time and a place for sharing concerns and discussing evidence that what someone is doing isn't working. But this approach works primarily if it is done in a relationship where the other person generally feels cared for and accepted.

Think about your own experiences with criticism and other negative interactions. How did these experiences make you feel about yourself and toward the other person? Sometimes arguments are necessary and healthy, but arguing shouldn't be your primary approach.

Fifth: Ask What the Person Would Find Helpful

Directly ask your friend or family member exactly what they would like you to do. What can you do that would be helpful? In what specific ways do they want you to help them?

Remember, you do not have to do something just because they ask you. On the other hand, if you don't ask or they don't tell, the two of you will find it hard to work together as a team.

In some ways helping someone is like being in a car with two drivers. If the drivers disagree on where to go or how to get there, one may be pushing the accelerator while the other is grabbing the emergency brake. You have to have minimal agreement about when and in what ways to help.

If the two of you don't agree on ways to help, use communication skills to try to resolve this disagreement. See Chapter 18: Communication Skills for suggestions.

If you still can find no way to help that is acceptable to you both, you may need to accept that, at this time or with this issue, there is no way you can help. Sometimes people just have to agree to disagree.

Consider whether there are additional factors to take into account when you communicate with your family member. Memory, concentration, and attention span can be affected by medications, medical conditions, psychological problems, or aging. Make sure you have realistic expectations about what a family member can understand and recall. You may need to adapt your communication style.

How Do I Deal With My Own Feelings?

It is natural to feel fearful, worried, or sad when you see your friend or family member dealing with lymphedema—especially if they are not managing their condition successfully.

Talk to them about your feelings. Start with listening to their point of view about the situation. Then try to help using the suggestions above.

You may want to read Chapter 3 on coping with sadness and grief, Chapter 5 on coping with fear, and Chapter 7 on coping with worry.

Specific techniques from Chapters 16-18, which include thinking skills, action skills, and communication skills, may also be helpful.

How Do I Deal With My Guilt Feelings

We can feel guilty for a number of reasons. We may have good reason for guilt and remorse. Sometimes we need to make amends or change. Sometimes we need to forgive ourselves for the past and work to change the present and future.

On the other hand, at times we feel guilt needlessly. It can be difficult to sort out how realistic our guilt feelings are and what we should do as a result. Guilt is uncomfortable emotion. Sometimes we respond by immediately denying any possible responsibility and assuming that the feeling guilt is unwarranted. Sometimes we go to the other extreme and immediately assume we are wrong.

Your feeling, by itself, isn't proof of either conclusion. You need to explore the assumptions you are making and what the facts are.

If you are feeling guilty, ask yourself these three questions:

- *"Have I done something in the past for which I have good reason to feel guilty?"* If the answer is yes, consider what you can do that will be appropriate and feasible:

  - Can you apologize or show remorse or sorrow?

  - Can you take action(s) to fix the consequences?

  - If you cannot change what happened, are there other ways that you can make amends?

  - What have you learned from what happened?

  - How will you use what you have learned in positive ways?

- *"Am I doing things currently in my life for which I have good reason to feel guilty?"* If the answer is yes, decide what and how you will begin to change:

  - What are you doing and why is it wrong or inappropriate?

  - What are the consequences of not changing? What will happen?

  - What are the benefits of changing? What will happen?

  - What specific things are you willing to do differently now so you can feel good instead of guilty?

- *"Am I feeling guilty about things that are (or were) wholly or partly out of my control?"* If the answer is yes, work to gain perspective on how much of what you feel guilty about is actually your responsibility:

  - If you are feeling guilty about things in the past, were your actions freely chosen or were other people or other factors responsible for your decisions and actions?

  - If you are feeling guilty about your friend or family member's decisions about lymphedema, remind yourself that you can only be responsible for those things that you directly control.

We can try to influence those we care about, but we don't control them. Because we do not have control over them, we cannot feel guilty or responsible for their decisions and actions and the consequences of those decisions or actions.

Helping a friend or family member with the physical or emotional effects of their lymphedema can be time-consuming. If you are actively involved on a day-to-day- basis, be sure to take care of yourself, too. You need to care for your own physical and mental health.[4]

If you are still feeling guilty, the exercises in Chapter 16: Thinking Skills may help.

How Do I Deal With My Anger, Impatience, or Frustration

If you find yourself feeling impatient, frustrated, or angry, explore the thoughts behind your feelings and ask yourself the questions below. Our emotions are powerfully affected by our thoughts. Anger is usually triggered by some other emotion, such as fear.

Step back and think about what you are saying to yourself. Sometimes we set ourselves up for anger by expecting ideal behavior. Life is not an ideal. Other people aren't perfect. Just because something is right doesn't mean things will happen that way. Just because a thing *ought to be* does not mean that it *is*.

Every time you refuse to accept imperfect reality, you are likely to feel disappointed, impatient, or angry. Expecting things to be different than they are because they 'should be' different is like continuing to run into a brick wall because the wall 'should not' be there. This is not an effective strategy!

Dealing with Anger, Impatience, Frustration Worksheet

Ask yourself, *"What am I telling myself that makes me angry, impatient, or frustrated?"* Write your answer in the left column of Worksheet 22-2 on page 363.

Now, ask yourself, *"Is what I am telling myself true?"* Do objective facts and evidence support it? Would an unbiased, uninvolved observer agree? Write your answer in the second column of worksheet 22-2.

Sometimes we face painful, frustrating situations that we cannot change. When you are facing a problem that is currently unsolvable, your job is to keep from adding more emotional distress to that which is inevitable. Life will give us enough problems. You don't want to add to them by talking to yourself in ways that don't help.

Ask yourself, *"Is what I am saying helpful?"* Write your answer in the third column of the worksheet.

Ask yourself, *"What am I feeling underneath my anger and frustration?"* Listen inside to your deeper feelings and thoughts. Anger is always a secondary emotion. If you pay attention, you can discover the real feeling underneath. Anger usually is a response to feeling fearful, threatened, or attacked. Write your answer in the fourth column of the worksheet.

Use the energy of anger to solve or change whatever is triggering your anger. Consider what you can tell yourself instead. Write your answers in the right hand column of the worksheet.

If you want to get angry, get angry at the problem, not the person. Getting angry feels good at the moment and can seem very powerful, but it has serious problems.

Getting angry is not necessary. A person can strongly disagree or set limits without anger.

Think about how your anger or impatience affects your relationship. Getting angry with someone is one of the most damaging and ineffective ways to help that person.

Using anger to change someone usually results in the other person only changing temporarily, or only changing when you are around. The other person often ends up putting more energy into lying or hiding than into changing. Even when anger results in a change, the change tends to be temporary unless the person finds another reason to continue it.

If you are committed enough to your relationship to be reading this chapter, you obviously care about the other person. Use that caring and commitment to learn more effective ways of helping—ways that will strengthen the relationship, not harm it. In particular, the skills in Chapter 18: Communication Skills, and in Chapter 4, Anger and Resentment, may help.

Worksheet 22-2: Dealing With Anger, Impatience, Frustration

What I Tell Myself That Makes Me Feel Angry, Impatient, Or Frustrated	Is It True?	Is It Help-ful?	Underlying Feelings	What I Could Tell Myself Instead?

Dealing with Disagreements

When you disagree with what your friend or family member wants, start by checking with them Is what you heard what the other person meant? Be specific. .

If you confirm that you understand what the other person wants, and you still disagree with them, explain the problem you have with their request. Explain how you see things differently. Are there facts that only one of you knows that would change the other person's opinion?

If you both understand each other's position and agree on the facts, but you still disagree, then negotiate. Use the communication skills above and from Chapter 18: Communication Skills. Make an alternative suggestion. What are you comfortable doing? What can you agree on? Is there some compromise that's acceptable to each of you?

If no agreement can be reached, you may need to agree to disagree. It may be that the other person is at a different stage in the process of change than you thought they were. (To understand about the various steps in the process of change, see Chapter 15, Planning to Change.)

Pitfalls to Avoid

So far, this chapter offered suggestions for things *to do*. This final section focuses on things *not to do*.

To avoid the pitfalls below, you need to find a balance between extremes. Nearly everything in life has a positive side and a negative side. Going too far in either direction creates problems. You are seeking the middle ground.

Don't Dismiss Lymphedema as Unimportant

One pitfall is to dismiss the demands of lymphedema as unimportant. You may find yourself thinking or saying things like:

- "Why do you have to take those precautions? Just skip them. After all, one time can't hurt."

- "Do you really have to spend all that time and money on those stupid garments and exercises and treatments?"

- "How come you're asking me to do this? Why can't you do it? You're just lazy. Lymphedema is just an excuse."

Do any of the above statements sound familiar?

If so, you may be missing crucial information or you may be allowing your own emotions to blind you to the legitimate demands and limitations that lymphedema imposes. For more information, talk with your family member's lymphedema therapist or see the books and websites listed under "Lymphedema" in the **Resources** section at the end of this chapter.

Chronic illness stirs up uncomfortable and unpleasant emotions in both the person who has it and in those around them. We don't like chronic illness or its demands.

One very human response to discomfort is to deny that there's a problem. We want it to go away. Maybe if we pretend it's not there, it won't be there! That would be so nice. Life would be like it was before.

This is tempting, but not helpful. Acknowledge that lymphedema care is important and that it is terribly burdensome. You need to support your friend or family member.

If you are finding it difficult to do this, do some exploring inside your thoughts and feelings. What uncomfortable emotions are you experiencing that may be triggering thoughts like the ones above? Are you feeling:

- Overwhelmed. If so, what is most overwhelming?

- Sad. If so, what makes you most sad?

- Angry or resentful. If so, what triggers your anger? What is underneath your anger?

- Scared. If so, what are your worst fears?

- Guilty or ashamed. If so, what are you blaming yourself for? Is it really your fault? Are you the only one responsible or do other people or factors play a part as well?

- Reacting to things from your past. If so, are the lessons you learned in the past helping you now? Are they appropriate now?

- Struggling with present stresses. If so, what are your sources of stress?

Read the earlier chapters in the book that deal with the specific emotional problem areas you are confronting. Consider reading the three chapters that present many generally useful skills (Chapters 16–18).

Don't Agree That Self-Management Isn't Worth Doing

Sometimes your friend or family member may feel hopeless and/or over-whelmed. They may become discouraged when, despite their best efforts, lymphedema continues to require a daily regimen of massage, compression, exercise, and skin care—and still there is swelling and discomfort. They may want to give up.

Indeed sometimes they may appear to have given up. They may have stopped wearing compression garments or following their daily self-management routine.

When someone you care about feels and acts this way, it can be easy for you to feel hopeless as well. As a caring family member or friend, you face a special challenge when the person you care about is not doing well.

On the one hand, you cannot directly change someone else's thoughts, feel-ings, or actions. You do not control anyone other than yourself. On the other hand, sometimes we can influence other people by what we say or do.

What can you do?

In a situation like this, your challenge is to maintain a balance between optimistic hope and realistic acceptance. You have to accept, deep down, that only the other person can decide whether or not to change. At the same time, you want to steadfastly remind yourself and them that change is always possible as long as we live.

You want to offer help and encouragement, while respecting that adults have the right to make their own decisions and choices, even if those decisions or choices are harmful. (Obviously, this does not apply if the person is a child or if the person is not mentally able to make decisions. We are talking here about a "competent" adult, in the legal sense of the word "competent.")

Don't agree that things are hopeless. We often underestimate ourselves. Don't automatically agree that they don't have the strength or the will to make changes and manage their condition. Maybe they just haven't done so yet.

Look at the facts. See if you can help them overcome any external obstacles. When they aren't doing lymphedema self-care because of a real physical or financial limitation (such as being unable to reach to do the bandaging or lacking the money for compression garments), help them problem-solve.

Look for help. Brainstorm about creative solutions. Remember that problems are never solved by giving up.

No one knows what the future may bring. Anyone who has been living with lymphedema for years will occasionally "hit the wall" and say, *"I've had it with this self-care routine - no more of this for me. Just let it swell."* These episodes often occur when other things are going wrong in their lives. Most people recognize the negative side of this attitude before the swelling gets out of control or an infection develops. Others tough it out until the situation is really bad and they have to start over again with intensive treatment. As a concerned friend or family member you want to maintain open lines of communication to help the person get back on track.

Don't Over-Emphasize the Negative

You want to offer realistic, positive support. Lymphedema *can* be lessened with professional treatment. However, an ongoing self-management program is essential. Painful emotions or unhelpful reactions, no matter long-standing, can improve with work.

You *don't* want to emphasize only the negatives and make your friend or family member feel overwhelmed or hopeless.

Sometimes well-meaning friends or family attempt to show empathy and support by saying things like:

- "I would hate so much to have lymphedema. Life wouldn't be worth living if I had to do that self-management every day, day after day! I don't know how anyone could possibly do this."

- "It must be AWFUL! How terrible!" "How can you stand it? I'd never show my face outdoors if I had this."

- "I'm so sorry you have this. This is horrible. It must be ruining your life."

Play back these comments in your head. Do you hear the relentless emphasis on the negative? Now replay comments you have made. Listen to yourself.

If you realize you are making similar comments, the first thing I want you to do is to congratulate yourself on your honesty in admitting it. You can't change a problem if you don't know, or won't admit, that it exists.

Next, make a commitment to continue to notice when you say such things. Determine that you will work hard to change now that you understand that such comments are unhelpful.

Soften your emphasis on the negative. Move to a more balanced perspective. Deliberately change what you say and think about lymphedema.

Deliberately change how you phrase things. See Watch Your Language in Chapter 16. Emphasize the other person's accomplishments, their self-care efforts, their courage, their abilities, etc. in the midst of adversity.

For example, statements like these are much more likely to be helpful:

- *"I am sorry you have lymphedema, but I am so proud of how you take care of yourself."*

- *"You really do a lot to keep yourself well and to minimize the symptoms."*

- *"I am impressed by how you take care of yourself. I am glad you are my (friend, wife, parent, child...)."*

From Negative to Realistically Balanced Positive Worksheet

To change what you think and say:

- Write comments you have made, or heard, that over-emphasize negative aspects in the left hand column of Worksheet 22-3.

- Now write one or more alternatives that are more balanced and positive while still realistic in the right hand column of the worksheet.

Worksheet 22-3: From Negative to Realistically Balanced Positive

Balanced, Positive, Realistic												
Emphasis On The Negative												

Resources

Lymphedema

Living Well With Lymphedema by Ann Ehrlich, Alma Vinje-Harrewijn, PT, CLT and Elizabeth McMahon, PhD. Lymph Notes, 2005.

Lymphedema: A Breast Cancer Patient's Guide To Prevention And Healing by Jeannie Burt and Gwen White. Publishers Group West, 1999.

Coping With Lymphedema by Joan Swirsky and Dianne Nannery. Avery Publishing Group, 1998.

www.LymphNotes.com - an online resource and support group for persons with lymphedema and their family members and for lymphedema therapists. It also provides information about lymphedema, treatment resources, and support groups.

www.lymphnet.org - website of the National Lymphedema Network, a nonprofit organization providing information about lymphedema, treatment resources, and support groups.

Other Topics

For more information about communication skills, see Chapter 18. For more information about any of the other specific emotions or challenges, see the relevant chapters or check the index.

Notes

1   Kornblith AB, Ligibel J: Psychosocial and sexual functioning of survivors of breast cancer. *Semin Oncol* 30(6): 799-813, 2003.

2   **Writing Out The Storm: Reading and Writing Your Way Through Serious Illness or Injury** by Barbara Abercrombie. St. Martin's Griffin, 2002. p. 144.

3   "Quality of Life of Breast Cancer Patients with Lymphedema" by Velanovich & Szymanski. *American Journal of Surgery*, March 1999, pg 184.

4   **American Medical Association Guide To Home Caregiving** edited by A. Perry, MD. John Wiley & Sons, 2001, pp. 174-185.

Chapter 23:
For Parents of Children with Lymphedema

Parenting any child can be a challenge at times. When your child has lymphedema, it adds another factor into an already complex and emotion-laden mix, especially if the lymphedema appears during adolescence.

This chapter is written for you— the parent of a child with lymphedema. The first part of the chapter focuses on parenting your child with lymphedema. Each child is unique. Needs vary with the child's temperament and with where that child is in the process of growing into adulthood.

The second part of this chapter focuses on recognizing and dealing with the emotional impact that your child's lymphedema has on you and the rest of the family. A child's chronic illness can bring positives with it as well as negatives. We'll talk about how to increase the one and minimize the other.

Your Child Is Unique

Each child is an individual. Let's review some of the factors that make your child unique. What is your child's temperament? Where is your child in the process of growing into adulthood?

Individual Temperament

We are born with a mix of nine general traits known as our "temperament." These traits are:

- Activity level

- Distractibility

- Intensity

- Regularity

- Sensory Threshold

- Approach/Withdrawal

- Adaptability

- Persistence

- Mood

Differences in these traits appear in the first few months of life. Many children fall in the middle range; some children fall at one end or the other. Each characteristic has advantages and disadvantages.

These personal characteristics tend to remain fairly stable throughout our lives. Taking your child's temperament into account will help you be a more effective parent.

Let's review these traits and how they may affect coping with lymphedema, especially if your child falls at one extreme or the other.

Activity Level

Some children are more physically active than average, move a lot, and have a high energy level. High-activity children will need your guidance to find safe outlets for their energy and to avoid activities that could be dangerous. They may have more trouble following lymphedema precautions. On the positive side, their muscle activity will help to move the lymph.

Low-activity children may need to be encouraged to move and exercise in ways that help the flow of lymph. They may also need encouragement to maintain a healthy weight and lifestyle.

Distractibility

High-distractibility children can be easily distracted when upset, which can make them more responsive to soothing. On the other hand, they can also be easily distracted from necessary scheduled self-care. They may also need more encouragement, structure, and monitoring to ensure that they remember and complete their self-management tasks.

Low-distractibility children may be more likely to complete lymphedema self-care once they get started.

Intensity

High-intensity children have strong, intense emotional responses, both positive and negative. High-intensity children may need more soothing and need more help in coping with their distress. Particularly as they enter the teen years, you need to be prepared to do a lot of listening while they vent. In general, they may benefit from a calmer approach by parents.

High-intensity children may get very upset by the challenges lymphedema brings. They can be demanding at times, but you generally know how they feel about things.

Low-intensity children, on the other hand, may react to feeling upset or sad by getting quiet. With low-intensity children, you need to watch for small cues or you may miss how they feel.

Even a little complaint from a low-intensity child may signal significant distress. Take their complaints seriously. You probably want to be more actively responsive.

Regularity

Some children have a very predictable internal schedule. You know when they are likely to be hungry or sleepy. If you have a child who is high on regularity, you can schedule lymphedema care around this schedule.

If you have a child who is unpredictable, you need to be more flexible. They're not trying to be difficult but their needs and energy level vary from day to day. Yesterday they may have been calm and ready to do lymphedema care. Today, at the same time of day, they may be tired, cranky, or hungry. Expect the unexpected and stay flexible.

Sensory threshold

Some children, from the moment they are born, are highly sensitive to physical stimuli: sound, touches, bodily sensations, etc. High-sensitivity children may be much more distressed by things like the physical sensations of lymphedema bandages or compression garments.

On the negative side, they may complain more. You may need a great deal of patience and empathy with them. On the positive side, they may be far more aware of their body's needs and able to spot and respond to early signs of lymphedema problems.

Low-sensitivity children are less bothered by sounds, smells, and other sensations. They may be easier in some ways. On the other hand, they may need more teaching and reminders when learning to monitor and care for their lymphedema. A daily routine of visually checking for lymphedema changes may be particularly important for them because they may be unaware of physical sensations that are early warning signs of problems.

Approach/withdrawal

Some children enjoy new situations or new people and go quickly and eagerly forward. Other children tend to hang back or withdraw and need more time to adjust and become comfortable in a new situation.

When faced with a change, slow-to-warm up children do better if you tell them about it ahead of time, if you give them more time and space when dealing with new situations or people, and if you gently and persistently encourage them to explore at their own pace. The good news is that they may be more prone to think before acting. This may help them follow lymphedema precautions.

When changing treatment centers or therapists, you might talk to your slow-to-warm child about the change beginning a few weeks in advance. Considering arranging to have your child visit the new center or meet the new therapist once or twice before actually going for a treatment.

Quick-to-approach children may find it easier to make friends and to reach out socially. This can be a real asset in minimizing the self-consciousness that can occur with lymphedema. On the more negative side, such children may be more vulnerable to peer-pressure or acting on impulse. You may need to spend more time and repetition when teaching them to think for themselves about important issues related to their health.

Adaptability

Adaptability refers to how easily a child adapts to changes or transitions, like changing routines or switching from one activity to another. Quick-to-adapt children easily adjust to transitions and changes, which can be a plus when dealing with lymphedema fluctuations.

Slow-to-adapt children are likely to be happier with a set routine. This can be a positive when it comes to carrying out the same self-care tasks day after day. On the other hand, they may get more upset when faced with flare-ups and changes.

Whenever possible, give slow-to-adapt children plenty of warning before changes of any kind and budget more time for transitions. When you can foresee transitions or changes, think ahead about ways to prepare your child to handle them. For example, you may give slow-to-adapt children a 10-minute warning, a 5-minute warning, and a 2-minute warning (or set a timer which rings at intervals) before they have to stop their current activity and begin lymphedema management. You may start talking to them several days in advance about what to expect if you know they will be seeing an unfamiliar healthcare professional or having a change in their normal treatment routine.

Persistence

Persistence reflects how long a child will pursue an activity or goal in the face of obstacles. High-persistence children can be seen as stubborn when they continue an activity that we want them to stop. It may be hard to get them to stop what they're doing and switch to doing their lymphedema care.

On the other hand, this trait can be seen as very positive when it leads them to patiently persevere with activities like homework, music practice, or sports practice. High-persistence children may have an easier time following through a daily lymphedema self-care routine.

Low-persistence children may need more encouragement, praise, and monitoring to make sure they continue to follow lymphedema routines. They will be more likely to become discouraged by the need for following a daily routine. Take this into account and compensate for it. You may need to give these children more support at older ages than a high-persistence child.

On the plus side, low-persistence children often learn to turn to other people for help with tasks. As a result, they may develop strong social skills. This is positive because social support can counter self-consciousness. In addition, turning to others for help can be positive when it comes to collaborating with healthcare professionals and seeking out support, information, and people to help them with parts of the care routine that they cannot perform for themselves.

Mood

Some children react to the world in a primarily positive, happy way. Such children are sometimes described as having "a sunny disposition." Optimistic children tend to overcome obstacles more easily.

Research, in general, suggests that an optimistic approach to life is associated with many positive outcomes.[1] At the same time, you don't want your child to be so unrealistically optimistic that they deny the dangers of not controlling their lymphedema.

A child who tends to be more sensitive to the negative aspects of life will need more frequent support and encouragement. Criticism may need to be gentle. This child may need more praise. You may want to emphasize the positive.

You want your child to find a balanced approach to lymphedema: taking the potential consequences of poor lymphedema care seriously, while focusing on the positive results of good care.

Stages of Development

You can see how temperament affects your child's reactions and behavior and how temperament affects what you child needs from you. Age also affects how we treat our children and how they respond.

What children can understand changes as they grow and mature. What they need from a parent also changes as they age. Children pass through some fairly predictable developmental stages in their growth into eventual adulthood.

The child psychologist, Erik Erikson, wrote about eight stages of development, five of which occur between birth and late adolescence. At each stage of development, he theorized that the child faces a basic task. Let's review these stages and how the basic task of each stage may affect parenting a child with lymphedema at that age.

Stage One: Basic Trust vs. Mistrust (birth-2 years)

In the first one to two years of life, your child mainly needs love and responsive care. You want to send a consistent message to children that they are safe and that their needs will be met. If your child needs lymphedema care during this time, you will provide it with as much loving comfort as possible.

Stage Two: Autonomy vs. Shame (18 months-4 years)

Around the time between 18 months up to 4 years old, the developmental task for children is learning that they are individuals, separate from their parents. They develop their own thoughts, ideas, wishes, and preferences. First, they express their desires through action and then, increasingly, through words.

The tantrums and "NO!" of this stage are indications of growing independence, initiative, and autonomy. As parents, you need to set limits and lovingly discipline your children.

You need to insist on their compliance with lymphedema care. At the same time, you want to support their pride in themselves and their right to their feelings (even when they can't have what they want).

This is the beginning of learning two important life lessons. The first is that we can have and express our own feelings, even when they are different from those we love. The second is that sometimes we have to do things that we don't want to do. Both lessons are very important. You don't want to skip either of them.

Stage Three: Initiative vs. Guilt (3 ½ - school-age)

From about three and a half years old to about when children start formal education, the developmental task for children is to learn to imagine, to cooperate, and to play with others. Children learn to lead as well as to follow.

During this stage, teach your child more about lymphedema care. Let your child be a "big boy" or "big girl." Let your child help with, or even take over, certain tasks like gathering supplies or putting things in the laundry. You want your child to develop pride and confidence.

Encourage your child to talk about their feelings about having lymphedema. Listen and accept their feelings.

Encourage them to talk about their ideas about why they have lymphedema. Give them facts they can understand. Correct misinformation. Some children worry that lymphedema is a punishment for something they have done or not done.

Beginning with this stage and continuing until your child is an adult, give them increasing amounts of information about lymphedema. Correct any misunderstandings or confusion. Answer their questions. Help prepare them for answering questions about lymphedema (see Communication Skills, Chapter 18). Teach them about lymphedema.

Stage Four: Industry vs. Inferiority (1st-9th grades)

From first grade to around ninth grade or so, children increasingly need to develop self-discipline. They learn to obey the rules and to follow a schedule. Obviously, these tasks fit right in with learning lymphedema self-care skills, precautions, and routines.

Teach your children as much as possible in the early years. Use lots of praise. Start by helping them, then move to prompting and supervising them, and finally move to letting the child be as independently responsible as possible for routine care. But don't become entirely uninvolved. Continue to monitor, support, and advise—but move more into the background.

Continue to help them become educated and knowledgeable about lymphedema. You want to set as firm a foundation as possible before the task of stage five begins.

Stage Five: Identity vs. Identity Diffusion (13-20 years)

The task of this stage is to develop a *consistent* and *positive* sense of self. Adolescents struggle to create a sense of themselves as separate from their parents. At one moment, teens may want to be close to their parents and reliant upon them, while at the next, they may seem to want be completely independent and separate. This can be a confusing and trying time for both parents and teens.

Primary lymphedema most commonly occurs during this developmental stage. As a result, teens have to learn to cope with lymphedema at a time when they are especially self-conscious, eager to look and act just like their friends, and vulnerable to peer-pressure.

Since the primary developmental task is to develop a consistent and positive self-identity, problems in this stage can take two forms. In the first, the adolescent is unable to develop a *consistent* sense of self. In the second, the adolescent develops an identity that is consistent and stable over time, but one which is *negative*. Examples are given below.

Adolescents may fail to develop a consistent sense of identity. As a result, in adulthood, they lack a stable sense of who they are. They may go from career to career, relationship to relationship, always trying to "find" themselves. Lacking a consistent, stable sense of self, they may find it particularly hard to follow a stable routine of lymphedema care day after day. They may veer between excellent self-care and self-neglect.

Sometimes adolescents develop a sense of identity that is consistent, but negative. Examples would be the adolescent who has a clear, consistent self-identity as the leader of a violent gang or the adolescent who develops a stable identity as "the failure." A consistently negative view of oneself is a weak foundation for good self-care.

From about thirteen to about twenty, your job as parents is to support your children emotionally as they struggle to develop a sense of who they are. You encourage their positive efforts and try to guide them so that they gradually become more responsible, more reliable, more consistent, and more independent.

They may "try on" different roles and behaviors. There may be times when, as parents, you're ready to tear your hair out and you wonder if your child will ever "grow up."

In general, adolescents develop a sense of who they are now as young adults by trying to be *different* from who they were as 'kids,' by finding ways to be *different* from their parents, and by trying to be *just like* their friends.

Adolescents who have had lymphedema since childhood may want to demonstrate that they're not kids any more by no longer following their lymphedema self-care routine. They may try to prove to you, and to themselves, that they don't have to do what you tell them to do and that they can make their own decisions about lymphedema care. They may want to look and act like their friends.

As parents, you want to look for ways in which they can be different from you that are separate from lymphedema care. Find ways to let them make as many decisions as possible about lymphedema care and take as much responsibility as possible, while agreeing with them on some way to monitor that they are not being harmed.

Offer them opportunities to educate themselves about their lymphedema. Encourage them to talk to other adults about lymphedema care. Adolescents accept guidance far more readily from a non-parent such as a healthcare professional, relative, teacher, or family friend.

As a parent, it can be frustrating or embarrassing to have your teenager turn to some other adult for the same information you are able to give them. Remember that they need to hear it from someone other than you and that by allowing this to happen, you are being a good parent.

Most adolescents are self-conscious. Developing lymphedema for the first time during adolescence can make this much worse. It can be painful for adolescents to feel, act, or look different from their peers.

You may want to look for a lymphedema exercise group, swim program, teen support group, online support group, counselor, or other source of support for your teenager.

Drop everything and listen when your teenager wants to talk. Be generous with praise, support, empathy, and encouragement. Encourage hope and problem solving.

If your young adult child goes away to college, discuss with your child what to do in case of infection or symptom worsening. Discuss how to monitor, where to get treatment, whether to carry antibiotics, and other key questions.

Plan ahead. At age eighteen, your child's medical information becomes private and can no longer be shared with you unless he or she signs a release of information permitting healthcare professionals to contact you. You and/or your child may want to educate college officials and student health center staff about lymphedema.

Successful Coping Is a Balancing Act

Children and adolescents may cope best with chronic illness if they:

- Accept help when appropriate, while also assuming increasing responsibility for self-care

- Find ways to rebel against and differentiate themselves from their parents that don't put themselves in danger

- Find satisfying activities to replace things they can't do because of lymphedema

- Can express a variety of feelings, for example, sadness or anger when they are frustrated and hope and confidence when things are going well

For some children, contact with other people who cope successfully with lymphedema is a powerful, positive experience and helps them develop confidence and optimism. Your lymphedema treatment facility may be able to help arrange this type of contact.

The Whole Family

Step back for a moment and think about your family as a whole. In a well-functioning family, the needs of any one child are balanced with the needs of all the other family members-children and adults.

Lymphedema affects the entire family. Lymphedema can bring positives. The siblings of a child with chronic disease can grow in maturity, responsibility, and empathy.

Lymphedema can bring negatives. Other siblings can feel as if they don't count or as if the ill child gets all the attention and love. They can feel that extra financial resources always get spent on the ill child. They can feel guilty or as if they have to put their needs on hold. This is particularly true if the child with lymphedema is hospitalized with a serious infection.

As a parent, you may be so aware of your child's needs that you don't take care of *yourself*. You need to keep yourself physically and emotionally healthy. Because of the stress of raising a child with a chronic condition, you need to make more effort to care for yourself than other parents.

If you also have lymphedema, you'll want to provide your child with a good role model in the way you handle your care and how you overcome the emotional challenges.

Finally, if you are married or in a long-term committed relationship, you want to nurture this relationship as well. Think about how you can balance meeting the needs of the child with lymphedema, the needs of other children or family members, your personal needs, and the needs of your relationship.

You and Your Family Are Unique

For better or for worse, our children stir up intense feelings from deep inside us. As parents, it is often in response to our children that we have some of the strongest feelings of selfless love, piercing regret, heart-stopping fear, angry frustration, and intense joy.

On the positive side, because of this intense emotional connection we may do things for the sake of our children that we might never do for ourselves. We may grow emotionally as we strive to meet their needs. On the negative side, the intensity of our feelings can lead us to say and do things that are not in anyone's best interest.

Our children are extensions of ourselves; yet they are unique, separate individuals. They will grow to make their own choices and create their own lives. Their independence is not rejection of us. In fact, it may be a validation that we have helped them develop the confidence to separate from us. We have to both hold on and let go.

We want to guide them, protect them, and lead them to a better future. We take pride in their successes. We can be embarrassed and feel ashamed or guilty when they fail. Yet we cannot treat them as if their decisions, triumphs, or failures are a kind of report card, publicly evaluating us as parents.

On the negative side, parenting a child with a chronic condition can be stressful. On the positive side, you can experience personal psychological growth. Plus, your stress level can diminish the more you view your situation as a challenge that you can handle. Take some time to consider the positives and the negatives of having a child with lymphedema as you read the next couple of pages.

The Positives

Mastering the challenges of raising a child with lymphedema can bring positives into your life. What follows is a partial list of some of those positives. Think about what other positive outcomes you have noticed or that you could create.

Closeness

Dealing with a chronic condition can build a special closeness among family members. The family has surmounted this challenge together and has remained intact. Family members may have a special depth of trust in one another. You may feel a special bond between you and your child.

Think about signs of closeness, trust, or empathy.

_____

Pride

By bringing challenges, lymphedema also brings opportunities for pride. We don't take pride in handling the easy things in life. We take pride in handling the tough ones.

Think about times when you feel proud of yourself, your spouse, your child with lymphedema, your other children or other family members, or other people involved with your child's care.

_____

Achievement

Think about some of the things you and/or your family have accomplished as a result of lymphedema. What has given you a sense of achievement or accomplishment?

☐ Gaining knowledge about lymphedema

☐ Learning lymphedema care skills

☐ Advocating for my child

☐ Seeing lymphedema symptoms improve

☐ _____

☐ _____

☐ _____

Communication

Because of lymphedema, you may have had to learn to speak up. You may have talked honestly about some of the most important issues in life.

Think of those times when you communicated effectively with your child, your spouse, other family members, childcare workers, healthcare professionals, or others. Think about communication skills you have used in the course of dealing with your child's lymphedema.

_____

_____

Confidence

In the course of coping with lymphedema, there are times when you rely on yourself, times when you rely on your child, and times when you turn to others.

When have you felt a justified sense of confidence and trust in yourself or in others? To whom can you turn and for what kinds of help?

_____

_____

Joy

Recall moments of joy. Chronic conditions can sometimes make us feel like life is all drudgery and problems. Refuse to give in. Seek out joy. Remember and cherish joyful feelings and experiences. Each one is a gift.

_____

_____

Appreciation

It is natural to focus on problems because problems get our attention and demand action. Yet problems and challenges can also deepen our appreciation of what we have. Review your life situation emphasizing appreciation.

What is there to appreciate about your child? Think about your child's talents, actions, or personal qualities. Think about the opportunities you have to show and share love and to grow in wisdom, knowledge, and strength.

_____

_____

What do you appreciate about your family and other people in your life and your child's life? Recall examples of help, support, or understanding.

_____

_____

Stop and list other things you can appreciate, such as sight, hearing, beauty, etc.

_____

_____

Increasing the Positives Worksheet

Use the worksheet on page 387 to rate the positive emotions or outcomes discussed above. Add any other positives you can identify that aren't listed here.

Rate each positive using the 0 – 10 scale. How strong is it? Write your answer in the second column of the worksheet.

How often does it happen? Write your answer in the third column.

Do you want that positive to happen more often? Mark Yes or No in the fourth column.

For each positive that you marked "Yes", plan what you'll do so that it happens more often and write your answer in the right hand column.

How do you feel about your plans to increase the positives in your life?

_____

If you are dissatisfied with your plans, consider reading Chapters 16-18 for ideas.

The Negatives

Now let's look at the other side. Step back and consider some of the negative feelings that you may experience in response to having a child with lymphedema.

Acknowledging negative feelings can be difficult, uncomfortable, or embarrassing. It is also the first step to changing them and protecting you and your family from any harm these feelings could otherwise cause.

Look at these feelings with some compassionate understanding. Each one of these negative emotions is understandable and natural. We all feel them at times.

Sadness and Grieving

When our child develops lymphedema, we grieve. We grieve the loss of the healthy child we had (or anticipated). We grieve for the impact on our child of having a chronic condition to be managed for life.

If a child develops secondary lymphedema due to an accident, cancer treatment, other medical procedure we have two challenges to overcome: grief over the initial incident and now lymphedema. Depending on what caused the child's lymphedema, you may want to read Chapter 4 for specific suggestions on dealing with anger.

We grieve for the loss of time that now must be spent caring for lymphedema. We grieve for the carefree innocence of not having a chronic condition.

The challenge presented by grief and sorrow is to find ways of working through these feelings that do not frighten or overwhelm your child. Write any suggestions that come to mind.

_____

_____

If you feel that you are stuck in sorrow or cannot move beyond your grief, read Chapter 3: Sadness and Grieving.

Worksheet 23-1: Increasing the Positives

Positives	How Strong 0 – 10	How Often? 0 – 10	Want More? Y/N	What I'll Do							
Closeness											
Pride											
Achievement											
Communication											
Confidence											
Joy											
Appreciation											

Pity

Pitying your children or seeing them as helpless victims is neither helpful nor useful. Your child needs your support and your love, not your pity.

Empathizing with your child's feelings and struggles is a loving response. Respecting their feelings is important.

Counter a negative, pitying view of your child by making a comprehensive list of your child's strengths, potential, skills, and positive traits. Add additional positives to the list as they occur to you.

_____

_____

Read the list over and over. Keep these factors in your mind whenever you think about your child or interact with your child.

Hopelessness

Children can overcome tremendous odds, especially if they feel someone cares about them and believes in them. Your view of your child and your child's future can be a self-fulfilling prophecy. Don't predict negatives.

If you are going to make predictions, predict success and hope. Hopeful, optimistic children and adults tend to be more successful and happier.[2] Write down some things you can say that are true and that convey hope and optimism.

_____

_____

If you are feeling generally negative, sad, or hopeless, read Chapter 5: Sadness and Grieving.

Fear

You may fear for your child's health and worry about the future. You may have thoughts such as, *"Am I doing everything I should do?", "Will my other children get it?" "Will the symptoms and demands of lymphedema hurt my child's self-image and quality of life?" "What's going to happen?"*

Like hopelessness, fear and worry are influenced by what we tell ourselves. Keep reminding yourself that you don't know the future. Also remind yourself that although lymphedema is a chronic condition, it is not malignant. Properly treated, lymphedema will not shorten the child's life.

You want to find the middle ground between unrealistic optimism on the one hand (*"Oh, don't worry. Lymphedema won't be a problem. You don't have to do self-care."*) and unrealistic pessimism and fear on the other (*"Disaster lurks everywhere. You can't cope now and will never learn to cope."*)

Your goal is to have an attitude of "realistic" fear and caution. You want your child to cope, not to cower. Look at what you just wrote. Write down anything else you want to say to your child to avoid unnecessary fear.

For more discussion of fear, read Chapter 5: Fear and Chapter 7: Uncertainty and Worry.

Overprotective

The reality is that you and your child do have to take protective actions and precautions that other parents and children don't. It can be easy to become over-protective, especially if you are feeling pitying, hopeless, and/or fearful.

You want to find a middle ground of realistic protection. The degree of protection you provide for your child should decrease as your child grows, especially in adolescence. The ways in which you provide that protection should also change as your child matures.

Write down your thoughts.

For more on this topic, read Chapter 6: Increased Self-Protection. If you aren't sure what appropriate self-protection is, talk to your child's healthcare professionals, read books such as **Living Well with Lymphedema,** and seek information from reputable sources. See **Resources** at the end of this chapter.

Guilt

You may feel guilty for your child's lymphedema, or for the demands it places on the family, or for the attention it takes from the other children. Your guilt may make it hard to set limits and discipline appropriately. Or it may interfere in your life and parenting in other ways.

If you are struggling with guilt, read Chapter 11: Asking "Why?"

When You Are Not At Fault

Sometimes people blame themselves when there is no realistic basis for blame or guilt. If you know this is true in your case, and yet you still feel guilty, focus on the facts.

- Did you deliberately and knowingly cause the lymphedema?

- Could you have absolutely predicted the result of your actions?

- Realistically, could you alone have prevented the lymphedema (or other problem about which you feel guilty)? Or is this a situation where other important factors, which are outside your control, also play a role and contribute?

Get all the facts you need to answer these questions. You need accurate information. For example, even when primary lymphedema runs in a family, the genetic risk is estimated at 50%, which means your child was just as likely *not* to inherit it. Primary lymphedema can occur unpredictably, for unknown reasons. As one pediatrician told a parent, *"It's a spontaneous mutation. Every disease started somewhere with a mutation."*

Write down the answers to the questions above or any other similar questions.

_____

_____

Review your answers. Find and review other relevant facts. Go over this information deliberately and repeatedly.

When You Think You Are At Fault

If you believe there *is* a realistic basis for your feelings of guilt, first stop and consider whether you may be depressed (see the checklist on page 37), because having and believing unrealistic, unfounded feelings of guilt commonly occurs with depression. Depression changes your thinking as well as your feelings and can make you believe things that are not true.

If there is even the slightest possibility that depression may be affecting you, consult a mental health professional. If you are depressed, get effective treatment.

If you are not depressed, but you still feel guilty and blame yourself, talk to someone who is knowledgeable, objective, and whose opinion you trust. This person should know all the facts about your child's situation and be knowledgeable about lymphedema.

If they say you are not responsible and should not feel guilty or to blame:

- Have them explain why.

- Write down what they say.

- Ask them to explain any confusing facts or logic until you understand it.

- Review this information as often as you need until your sense of guilt diminishes.

- If, despite the facts, you are still convinced you are responsible, consider getting professional psychological help with this issue.

Reality-Based Guilt

If the objective, knowledgeable person agrees that you *are* to blame, consider seeing a psychotherapist to address this issue. Guilt can trigger positive actions or it can be destructive.

If you are dealing with reality-based guilt, consider these points:

- Wallowing in guilt helps no one, fixes nothing, and leads to no positive change. Your guilt does not help your child, your family, or the lymphedema.

- Remorse can be positive when it leads to corrective actions, such as making amends either to the person involved or in some other way.

- Acknowledgement of realistic guilt can be positive when it leads to change. For example, if your young child's lymphedema worsens when you skip their home care treatment, guilt may help motivate you to problem-solve so home treatment improves.

- Acceptance of guilt can be positive when it can lead to forgiveness— from others or from yourself.

- For your child, if not for yourself, you must find the strength to rise above guilt and make a more positive future.

Write down any ideas you have.

_____

_____

Review Chapter 11: Asking "Why?" and use the techniques in Section IV: Tools for Change.

Blame

The ideas and suggestions you just read about guilt and blaming yourself apply to blaming others.

If you are blaming someone else for your child's lymphedema, ask the questions above about the person(s) you blame. Write the answers to these questions here.

_____

If you are struggling with blame, read both Chapter 11: **Asking "Why?"** and Chapter 4: **Anger and Resentment.**

Anger

Anger can be helpful when it gives us the energy, commitment, and perseverance to make positive change. But even in these circumstances, anger is less helpful than determination and persistence.

You may find yourself getting angry at things you can't change, like the past, other people, or genetics. For example, you may be angry when your child fails to follow self-care recommendations. Ask yourself "What positive purpose does anger serve then?"

Anger can eat you up inside, destroy your relationships, and even damage your health. Ask yourself: *"Is it is really worth it?"* Write the answers to these questions here.

_____

Anger can distract us from the real issue or feelings that need to be addressed. We may be feeling angry as a defensive reaction to underlying, painful emotions that are the real problem.

Acting on our anger can keep us from identifying and dealing with the real problem. You may find yourself feeling angry at the child with lymphedema or at your spouse because anger is a protection from other painful emotions like the ones discussed earlier in this chapter.

If you are struggling with anger, carefully read Chapter 4: **Anger and Resentment.**

Overwhelmed

Consider whether you may be trying to do too much. Ask yourself:

1. What really *must* be done?

2. What can be postponed, or done by someone else, or done less often, or done more quickly or less thoroughly?

Consider whether you may be struggling with depression.

Consider whether feeling overwhelmed is a signal that you need more support, less stress, or that there are problems in your life that you need to address. Are there practical problems such as time management, finances, childcare, or health insurance that need solutions? Write the answers to these questions here.

_____

_____

Read Chapter 2: Feeling Overwhelmed.

Decreasing the Negatives

Use worksheet 23-2 on page 395 to rate each of the negative emotions or reactions discussed above. Add any other negative emotions or reactions you identify.

Rate the strength of each emotion using the 0 – 10 scale in the second column.

How disruptive is it? Rate it on a scale of 0-10 in the third column.

Do you need to change it? Mark Yes or No in the fourth column.

For each emotional reaction where you marked "Yes" under Need to Change, rate how ready you are to change it and how confident you are that you'll succeed in changing in the fifth and sixth columns.

Now make your priority list. Decide which emotions you will work on changing first, then second, and so on. Write your answers in the right hand column.

Later in this chapter you'll develop a plan for making these changes.

When to Seek Professional Help

Negative emotions can cause waves of intense distress. But the frequency, intensity, and duration of the distress should gradually subside over a few weeks or months. You should be able to function despite your distress.

Seek professional help if you notice *any* of the following. You feel strong negative emotions and they:

- Are not lessening at all in any way after several weeks.

- Are very strong and intensely distressing all the time for more than a few days.

- Interfere significantly with your ability to function.

- Leave you unable to experience any pleasure or enjoyment.

- Interfere significantly in your relationships with other people.

Worksheet 23-2: Decreasing the Negatives

Negative Emotion	How Strong 0 – 10	How Disruptive? 0 – 10	Need to Change? Y/N	Ready to Change? 0 – 10	Able to Change? 0 – 10	Priority
Grief						
Pity						
Hopelessness						
Fear						
Overprotective						
Guilt						
Blame						
Anger						
Overwhelmed						

Nurturing a Positive View of Your Child

Your view of your child and of your child's future influences *your child's* self-view and view of the future.

Realistic Optimism

Strive for an attitude of realistic optimism:

- Acknowledge the negatives.

- Work to decrease the negatives or to minimize their impact.

- Identify and emphasize the positives.

- Work to increase the positives and to increase both your own and your child's awareness of the positives.

How do you think about and talk about your child and your child's future? Are your views ones that you would be pleased to have your child take inside and use as guides?

Three Pitfalls to Avoid

How we think about our children shapes the way we interact with them. Here are three pitfalls to avoid in how you think about your child.

Helpless Victim

Children are lovable and helpless when they are born. They depend on us for everything. We want to protect them from all danger, harm, or rejection.

When our child is diagnosed with a chronic condition, it naturally intensifies or reactivates this feeling, at least temporarily. We can fall into the trap of emphasizing our child's vulnerability.

We can view our child as a helpless victim. This does no one any good.

Your child will have to deal with lymphedema for the rest of his or her life. You want your child to feel competent and able. Foster that view in yourself, in others, and in your child.

Explicitly praise the ways in which your child is competent and able. Predict aloud to your child that she or he will become even better at dealing with lymphedema as she or he grows older and more mature. Do this often.

Mirror of Yourself

"She has my nose." "He has my eyes." We look for ways that our children are like us. We feel a deep connection and commitment to our children and, in fact, we often do share likes, dislikes, or temperament traits.

These similarities can blind us to the ways in which our children are different from us. The truth is that our children are not identical to us, no matter how close we are.

Your child may not view lymphedema the way you do. Your child may cope differently, react differently, think differently, and feel differently. What your child needs from you may be different from what you would need or what you needed at that age. Listen and respond to your unique child.

As a Parental Report Card

Because our children are unique individuals, they will inevitably make choices with which we disagree. And yet, think how often people react as if a child's choices or actions are a kind of parental "report card."

We tend to take (or be given) credit for our child's successes. We tend to blame (or be blamed for) their failures. This way of thinking sets you up to have more negative feelings, such as fear, guilt, blame, and anger.

If you find yourself thinking this way, fight back by considering this logically:

- Both you and your child are doing the best you can.

- You are separate individuals.

- Your child's successes and failures are their own, not yours. Their choices in how they deal with lymphedema and respond to situations are theirs, not yours.

When problems arise, look for solutions. But don't take the ups and downs personally. Having a child with lymphedema is challenging enough. You don't have to carry a burden of feeling invalidated as a person when things aren't perfect.

Nurturing a Positive View of Your Child's Future

Regardless of our intent, what we say about our child's future can act as a self-fulfilling prophecy. Things we say during moments of fear or exasperation may be repeated in our child's mind for years to come.

How do you think about and talk about your child's future? Would you want these words to shape your child's view of the future or themselves?

You don't want negative, fearful words shaping your child's view. You want positive, realistic, coping words guiding your child's actions.

Avoid Over-Emphasizing the Negative

As parents, part of our job is to look ahead and see potential problems so that we can help our children avoid them. The danger is that we can over-emphasize the negative.

Do you expect that your child will be unhappy? Alone? Socially-isolated? Self-conscious? Unable to cope with lymphedema?

Do you find yourself frequently talking to your child about problems? Are you focusing on disasters narrowly avoided or looming ahead? Are you warning your child about possible mistakes too often?

These can all be signals that you are over-emphasizing the negative.

Avoid Being Unrealistically Positive

Being unrealistically positive is the other extreme. Not caring for lymph-edema leads to harm. You can't tell your child it doesn't matter whether or not they follow self-protection and self-care guidelines because it *does* matter!

At the same time, lymphedema can fluctuate even with ideal care. And no one is perfect – especially while they are growing up.

Accidents happen. Even the most responsible child is unlikely to always follow self-care guidelines. If you never expect problems, you and/or your child will be more distressed when problems occur.

You don't want to predict a total absence of problems. You want to predict that your child will find ways to learn from problems and to cope with them. This is how children develop skills, knowledge, and resilience.

Finding a Balance

Finding a balance is a core theme throughout this chapter and this book. Think about your child's life, your family's life, and your own life.

Check the areas where you are pleased with the balance you have achieved. Congratulate yourself.

☐ Emphasizing lymphedema care vs. emphasizing child's strengths, activities and interests

☐ An emphasis on safety and avoiding danger vs. an emphasis on having fun and encouraging adventure and exploration

☐ Meeting the needs of the child/children with lymphedema vs. meeting the needs of the others in the family

☐ Focus on the child vs. focus on yourself and your partner

If there are areas where you want a better balance, make a note of them and write down any ideas you have here.

_____

_____

Taking Action

Review Worksheet 23-1: Increasing the Positives. Review the actions you will take to increase the positives. Write down any other ideas that come to you now.

_____

_____

Changing the Negatives Worksheet

Think about the ideas in this chapter and your answers to the various questions and worksheets, especially Worksheet 23-2: Decreasing the Negatives.

Look at your top priorities and write down some specific actions you'll take to decrease the negatives in the worksheet on page 401.

The Next Step

Now that you have identified changes you want to make, follow these steps:

- Read Section IV: Tools For Change
- As you work to make changes, you may wish to reread this chapter.
- Redo the worksheets to see your progress over time.
- For more general information on parenting, see the books listed below.

Thank you for reading this chapter - and congratulations. Take a moment to praise and support yourself. The fact that you are reading this says something very positive about you as a parent. You care enough about your child to seek information about effective parenting.

I hope the information in this chapter has been useful to you. I sincerely wish you and your family all the best.

Resources

Parenting

Parenting Through Crisis: Helping Kids In Times Of Loss, Grief, And Change by Barbara Coloroso. Harper Collins, 2000.

How To Talk So Kids Will Listen And Listen So Kids Will Talk by Adele Faber and Elaine Mazlish. Avon Books, 1999.

Kids, Parents, and Power Struggles by Mary Kurcinka. HarperCollins, 2000.

The Optimistic Child: A Revolutionary Program That Safeguards Children Against Depression & Builds Lifelong Resilience by Martin Seligman, et al. Houghton Mifflin, 1995.

Raising Your Spirited Child: A Guide for Parents Whose Child Is More Intense, Sensitive, Perceptive, Persistent, Energetic by Mary Kurcinka. Perennial, 1998.

Worksheet 23-3: Changing the Negatives—Taking Action

Negative Emotion	Priority	What I'll Do To Decrease The Negative
Grief		
Pity		
Hopelessness		
Fear		
Overprotective		
Guilt		
Blame		
Anger		
Overwhelmed		

The Preventive Ounce (as in *"An ounce of prevention is worth a pound of cure"*) website (www.preventiveoz.org) offers free, interactive questionnaires to help you identify your child's temperament. The questionnaires are designed for children from 4 months up to 5 years old and will be most useful to parents of children younger than four years old.

Temperament Tools by Helen Neville and Diane Clark Johnson. Parenting Press, 1997.

Lymphedema

Living Well With Lymphedema by Ann Ehrlich, Alma Vinje-Harrewijn, PT, CLT and Elizabeth McMahon, PhD. Lymph Notes, 2005.

www.LymphNotes.com – an online resource and support group for persons with lymphedema and their family members and for lymphedema therapists. It also provides information about lymphedema, treatment resources, and support groups.

www.lymphnet.org – website of the National Lymphedema Network, a nonprofit organization providing information about lymphedema, treatment resources, and support groups.

Notes

1   **The Optimistic Child: A Revolutionary Program That Safeguards Children Against Depression & Builds Lifelong Resilience** by Martin Seligman, et al. Houghton Mifflin, 1995.

2   **The Optimistic Child: A Revolutionary Program That Safeguards Children Against Depression & Builds Lifelong Resilience** by Martin Seligman, et al. Houghton Mifflin, 1995.

Chapter 24

For Healthcare Professionals

This chapter is for all healthcare providers who see patients with lymphedema. The ideas presented will be particularly relevant when diagnosing or treating lymphedema, but they are designed to be helpful whether or not lymphedema is the focus of your treatment.

What Lymphedema Means Physically

You may already understand the basic facts about lymphedema:

- Lymphedema is a serious chronic condition that can be painful, disfiguring, and disabling.

- Lymphedema is a relatively common consequence of the surgical treatment of cancer, especially breast, gynecologic, genitourinary cancers, melanoma, and sarcoma. Its incidence increases over time.[1][2]

- Swelling due to the accumulation of lymph causes the affected limb, or area, to be enlarged, heavy, and misshapen. This can result in visible disfigurement, impaired function, pain, orthopedic problems, limited mobility, and disability.

- Unless controlled, lymphedema will progress. Fibrosis, hyperkeratosis, and papillomatosis may develop.

- For patients with lymphedema, even the smallest break in the skin places them at risk of developing infections such as cellulitis. If the infection is penicillin resistant or if the patient is diabetic, allergic to antibiotics, or immune-compromised, treatment may require hospitalization and intravenous antibiotics.

- Lymphedema can usually be controlled through ongoing treatment, but this may mean a lifelong regimen of daily compression, exercises, self-massage, and specialized skin care.

To learn more about the physical aspects of lymphedema and lymphedema care, see Appendix A and the resources listed at the end of this chapter.

What Lymphedema Means Emotionally

“ Lymphedema is a chronic and debilitating disease....It generally is under reported and under treated. The effects of lymphedema on a patient's quality of life are substantial and can be devastating.[3] ”

The forms of lymphedema commonly seen in the North America are primary and secondary lymphedema.

Primary lymphedema is often an inherited condition. Swelling can result from malformation or deficiency of the lymphatic vessels. This condition can appear, without warning, at any age. Some primary lymphedema patients have been coping with it since birth. Most cases of primary lymphedema develop during puberty and affect the feet and legs, with a higher incidence in females than males. Puberty is an emotionally stressful period for most people. Developing lymphedema during this time can be especially upsetting for patients who are sensitive about their weight or appearance.

Secondary lymphedema is caused by damage to the lymphatic system as result of surgery, radiation, burns, or other trauma. A significant percentage of cancer survivors develop it as a consequence of treatment, especially treatment for breast cancer, prostate cancer or melanoma. Onset is often delayed and those who are at risk for lymphedema will remain at risk for the rest of their lives. Incidence increases with each year post-treatment.

Secondary lymphedema carries an additional emotional burden when the condition results from medical treatment. When this is the case, it can complicate relationships between the patient and all medical professionals.

Patients Can Feel "Stuck" and Angry

Secondary lymphedema is a constant reminder of the injury, illness, or medical procedure that was its cause. Because they must deal with lymphedema every day, it is harder for patients to put the past medical trauma behind them and go on with their lives.

Not uncommonly, breast cancer survivors say that having lymphedema is harder for them to deal with emotionally than having breast cancer. Many individuals with secondary lymphedema feel angry and betrayed by the medical profession when the lymphedema is the result of a diagnostic or treatment procedure.

Many patients report that they were never informed of the possible risk of lymphedema before agreeing to the medical procedure that caused it. Justifiably or not, they feel they were harmed in the course of procedures done to help them—and now they are left with a condition that has no cure.

Understandably, they can feel angry, betrayed, and abandoned. They may find it hard to trust anyone associated with healthcare. Even if you had nothing to do with the original cause of the lymphedema, feelings remain that impact your relationship with the patient.

Lymphedema Can Be Emotionally Tiring and Stressful

Because it is a chronic condition, lymphedema can't be ignored or forgotten. It must be actively treated and managed daily for the remainder of the patient's lifetime.

Lymphedema interferes with simple pleasures and activities that most of us take for granted such as taking a long soak in a hot bath. Patients must guard against 'overuse' or anything that would increase swelling. Because of the danger of infection, the patient must always be alert for anything that may break or puncture the skin. Anyone with lymphedema—or at risk of developing lymphedema—is cautioned to wear a compression garment when traveling by air.

People get tired of the daily self-management routine. Patients long for a respite from this ongoing battle. Some become sufficiently discouraged that they give up on self-care and stop taking necessary precautions. This can result in serious infections. Lymphedema may worsen to the point where it can no longer be ignored. Irreversible damage may result.

The effects and demands of lymphedema can create stress for the patient's family as well. As a result, family members may be less able to offer emotional support to your patient.

Care Is Time-Consuming, Expensive, and Not Reimbursed

Effective lymphedema care includes treatment and self-management as explained in Appendix A. Treatment ranges from intensive inpatient programs to periodic therapist visits. Typically the lymphedema therapist will teach the patient about self-management and monitor their progress. Responsibility for most of the day-to-day care rests on the patient and family.

Self-management includes self-massage, specialized exercises, the constant use of compression garments or bandages, and skin care. These activities may take up to two or more hours each day. Many patients require assistance with some aspects of their self-management.

Medicare and most health insurance companies do not cover all the costs associated with lymphedema management. Many do not reimburse the cost of compression garments or bandages. Therefore your patient has ongoing out-of-pocket expenses.

Some patients must forego necessary, physician-ordered treatment because insurance does not cover the costs of treatment and the patient cannot afford to pay for it. Many patients are forced to spend additional time and energy fighting for insurance coverage or reimbursement of professional treatment sessions.

People Can Feel Lonely, Frightened, and Abandoned

Your patient may have had to cope with lymphedema symptoms on their own for many years, without appropriate knowledge or guidance because the condition was not diagnosed, treatment was not available, or they could not afford treatment.

Some patients, particularly those with primary lymphedema, may have been symptomatic for many years before receiving a diagnosis. During this time, they lacked both effective treatment and emotional support from others facing the same condition.

Many people with lymphedema complain that they were never warned about the possibility of lymphedema. They were not told about its early warning signs nor advised on precautions to help prevent it. And when they do develop, its impact is dismissed.

> **"** *My doctor told me nothing about what could happen. When I got lymphedema, I asked him, 'How come you didn't warn me?' And you know what he says, ' You had so much on your plate that I [unilaterally] decided you couldn't absorb any more.' I told him, 'That's ridiculous.' So now here I am—just finished ten days in the hospital on antibiotics for cellulitis. All he says to me is, 'Well, you don't have cancer any more.'* **"**

They also report that their healthcare providers have little to offer them once the condition is diagnosed. This can be because the professional has little experience with lymphedema or because their training covered diagnosis but not treatment. For example, after making the diagnosis, a physician may write a prescription for treatment by a trained lymphedema therapist—but not make specific recommendations about where, or how, to find such a therapist. This leaves much of the burden on the patient and their family.

Outside the healthcare field, most people have never heard of lymphedema and have no understanding of the lymph system. This makes it hard to discuss the condition with others and find sympathy and support.

People talk about breast cancer and other cancers. National fund-raisers are given a lot of media publicity. Cancer survivors are lauded. Who talks about lymphedema? As one Lymph Notes member put it, *"Lymphedema feels like a dirty little secret because no one talks about it."*

People Feel Self-Conscious

A limb affected by lymphedema can swell to twice its normal size or more. Severe swelling can make the tissues hang in folds. Lymphedema is often visibly disfiguring. People with lymphedema may not be able to wear their normal clothing. Clothes may need to be large and baggy around the rest of the body in order to fit over the lymphedematous limb. This results in feelings of self-consciousness and can leave the person with a poor self-image.

The special compression garments or bandages that must be worn daily are bulky, uncomfortable, and visible. This leaves the patient struggling with physical discomfort while feeling self-conscious and, perhaps, ugly. Someone with lymphedema may be unable to keep it private and may often have deal with questions from strangers who can immediately see that something is wrong.

Lymphedema patients may also be self conscious about the way they move. They can be limited in their movements due to the weight of the swelling or due to orthopedic problems either caused or exacerbated by the lymphedema.

Also, secondary lymphedema can result from causes that, themselves, create self-consciousness and concerns about appearance. Two examples of this are lymphedema resulting from mastectomy surgery or from serious burns.

Quality of Life is Affected

There is no question that lymphedema negatively affects the quality of life.[4] Some patients with multiple conditions report that lymphedema has a more negative effect on their quality of life than other conditions. For example, a Lymph Notes member with multiple sclerosis, lupus, and primary lymphedema in both legs reports that "*I think the primary lymphedema is the most debilitating of all of these.*"

The results of a study of women after breast cancer treatment support the effect on quality of life. Those who developed lymphedema were compared with those who did not. Women with lymphedema reported more emotional distress and a lower quality of life, especially immediately after diagnosis and during intensive lymphedema treatment.

On the other hand, the news is not entirely negative. Quality of life scores improved after women completed intensive lymphedema treatment. In particular, improved scores were more frequent among those women who maintained their self-care plan after intensive treatment.[5]

Summary

Your patients with lymphedema will be dealing with difficult emotions. They may be angry and resentful. They may feel mistrustful and betrayed. They may find it hard to trust any healthcare provider.

Patients may feel anxious, frightened, and vulnerable. They may find themselves focusing on their body, fearing that any change is a sign of catastrophe. After all, they have already had one (or more) catastrophe.

People with lymphedema may feel abandoned by their healthcare providers, by their insurance, and/or by other people. They may feel worthless, isolated, and lonely.

They may feel stressed, discouraged, and overwhelmed. They may feel hopeless and like giving up.

What This Means for Your Patient Relationship

Emotions matter. These understandable, distressing, and difficult emotions can interfere with your relationship with your patient.

A strained relationship with your patient feels bad to both you and your patient. It impairs your effectiveness. It can make you doubt yourself. When your patient is unhappy with you, or when there is poor communication between you and your patient, you can both feel like you are failing.

Your patient may believe that you do not understand or that you don't care enough. This is personally unsatisfying to both of you. Plus, these factors are associated with a higher likelihood of malpractice suits.

Negative emotions generally make people less willing or able to carry out treatment recommendations—and faithfully carrying out recommended self-management is essential to good lymphedema care.

Apart from this, chronic emotional distress is strongly associated with poor health outcomes overall.

Responding to Your Patients' Negative Emotions

You may have been given generic advice about the importance of *"conveying empathy," "fostering a strong doctor-patient relationship," "having a good bedside manner,"* etc. However, few professionals are given specific suggestions for achieving these laudable goals.

If you were very lucky, you had may have had the opportunity to observe and learn from a skilled mentor. Chances are, though, that you may not have received much training or practice in effective communication.

Here are specific suggestions that will reduce your patient's negative emotions and your own. Interactions should become more effective and more rewarding. Try them out for yourself and see the results.

See It from Their Side

Step back and look at what your patients are dealing with. Is it any wonder they are emotionally upset?

They have a chronic, disfiguring, uncomfortable condition. They may have few sources of support. They may feel betrayed by the medical profession because medical treatment gave them this condition, because they weren't warned about it or told how to avoid it, or because health care offers no cure. Their health insurance or Medicare almost certainly doesn't cover all the related expenses.

Imagine how you would feel if you were in their shoes. View their emotions and reactions from their perspective.

Assume There Is a Reason for Every Reaction

Even the most destructive emotions or actions have reasons behind them. We all react based on our personality, our genetics and biochemistry, our past experiences, our expectations, and our knowledge or assumptions.

You can deal more calmly and effectively with your patients if you accept that there are reasons behind their reactions. You want to respect and try to understand their reasons.

Understanding does not mean liking, or agreeing with, or supporting. It just means understanding.

Sometimes people react the way they do because they are not yet ready to take action on a problem. If you know where someone is in the process of change, you are more likely to be able to understand them and help them progress.

Chapter 15: **Planning To Change** explains the five predictable stages in the process of any change. It covers how to identify where a person is in the process and what types of actions fit each step. You may find it very useful for helping change the behavior of patients who are having trouble with self-management or compliance.

Be Curious

Be curious when a patient surprises or frustrates you. Ask for information.

Use words that are neutral and non-blaming or that present your question as a request for help or clarification. Be generous in assuming your share (or more) of the lack of agreement.

Look for a way to make sense of what is happening. In particular, look for a way of understanding the other person that either leads to a positive action or at least protects the relationship and leaves a door open for change in the future. Try questions like:

- *"What are you feeling about ….?"*

- *"I am surprised by what you said/did. Tell me more so I can understand."*

- *"I would like to see this from your point of view."*

- *"Help me understand how you are feeling/how you see things."*

- *"What would you like from me if this were an ideal world and anything were possible?"*

Especially ask questions like this when your patient is angry with you. The natural reaction is to close the topic as soon as possible. The most effective response is the opposite. Be curious. Explore.

- *"What is making you angry?"*

- *"What else are you angry about?"*

- *"What else is there about this that angers or upsets you?"*

You will find it uncomfortable to explore disagreements and feelings like anger. Remind yourself continually of the benefits to you and your patients of doing this.

Being genuinely curious about your patient's reactions helps your patient become assertively honest and direct in their communication with you. This is good for your working relationship. It improves the quality of the information you receive, which improves the quality of the treatment plans you formulate.

Patient understanding and compliance with treatment recommendations will increase. Trust and patient satisfaction increase. Research shows that people with chronic conditions who are more specific and assertive with their health care providers have better outcomes.[6]

Communication Skills—What

The best advice in the world is useless if a poor relationship with you prevents your patient from following it. A positive working relationship is established and maintained by good communication. Good communication begins with understanding, acceptance, and respect.

Understand, Confirm, Accept

Your **first** step is to try to understand your patient. Your **next** step is to confirm that you understand correctly. Your **third** step is to show that you accept your patient's feelings and point of view with respect and empathy.

These three steps strengthen the relationship, clarify the issues, and increase the chances that your patient will listen to what you say. After all, aren't we all far more willing to listen and give credence to someone else if we feel understood and accepted by them first? If you contacted a consultant who didn't listen or understand what you were saying, would you trust their advice?

1. Summarize:

- *"So from where you sit, it seems as if ….."*
- *"As I understand it, you think or feel …"*

2. Check Your Understanding:

- *"Is that right?"*
- *"What have I misheard?"*
- *"Is there anything you've told me that I haven't understood?"*

3. Temporarily Step Over To Their Point of View:

- *"I can see how you would feel that way."*
- *"That must be very difficult for you."*

Respond

The **fourth** step in communication is to respond. Sometimes you can do what your patient wants. Sometimes you can't.

If You Can Do What They Want

Great. Do it.

Sometimes we just didn't understand what someone wanted. We didn't ask. They didn't say. We made the wrong assumptions.

Thank them for letting you know. Remember, you not only want to solve the immediate problem, you want to develop trust and honest communication.

If You Can't Do What They Want

Say so honestly while respecting their reasons for asking.

- *"I can see that it would be useful if ...., unfortunately, I can not (for these reasons)."*

- *"I understand how hard it is that we can't ....."*

- *"I know. It would be really nice if..... I'm sorry. We try to do the best we can and it's frustrating when we can't ...."*

Negotiate respectfully. Ask them what would be most helpful to them at this point given the constraints of reality.

- *"What would help instead?"*

- *"What can we do together that would be most useful to you at this point?"*

Offer an alternative.

- *"I can't .... Would it be helpful if I ...... or ....?"*

- *"I am not able to ...., but I can .... Would that be helpful to you?"*

Communication Skills—How

How we say something can be almost as important as what we say. And it can have an even larger effect of how (or if) the message is received.

Emphasize What Can Be Done

With everything in life, you can emphasize what *can* be done. Or you can emphasize what *can not* be done.

Emphasizing what can be done leads to more hope and action. This is especially important for chronic, challenging problems, like lymphedema. Emphasizing what cannot be done can create hopelessness, despair, and giving up.

What do I mean? Here are some examples:

- *"First of all, this is not a return of the cancer."*

- *"It is a chronic condition that can wax and wane. But I want you to know that, with proper treatment, it will not inevitably get worse."*

- *"While there isn't a cure, there are treatment. I will do everything I can to help you find them."*

- *"This can be controlled."*

- *"There are things you can do to help this condition. In fact, treatment and regular self-care can make a huge difference."*

Now listen to these counter-examples and hear the difference:

- *"There's no cure. You'll have it until you die."*

- *"There's nothing we can do. It's a permanent disease and it can get worse."*

- *"You will just have to learn to live with it Anyway you should be glad it's not cancer. At least you're not dead. Aren't you grateful for that?"*

To successfully treat and control lymphedema, patients have to be unceasingly vigilant. They must take precautions. They need to spend time, money and energy on treatment and self-management.

To succeed with lymphedema, your patients have to keep themselves motivated. They have to believe that maintaining self-management is both doable and worthwhile.

You want successful, healthy patients. Who's going to be more successful: a patient who feels hopeful and supported while facing a challenging but important task? Or a patient who feels hopeless and abandoned? Your word choice makes a difference.

Use Neutral or Positive Words

Listen to your words and how you think. Honesty is not the same as negativity. Emphasizing the positive is not the same as dismissing.

Do you describe, or think of, lymphedema as *devastating, hopeless, awful,* or *incurable*? Do you trivialize is as *just a little swelling, a minor inconvenience,* or *not a big deal*?

Or do you describe, and think of, lymphedema as *challenging, important to control,* and a *condition that can be controlled*. See Watch Your Language in Chapter 16 (page 246) for more examples.

Speak to the Specific Person

Speak so the person understands. Pitch your explanations to their level of knowledge. Use the words they use. Use concepts they understand. Think about what your words imply to them.

Address the other person's concerns. Speak to what's important to them. Different people are concerned about different aspects of lymphedema. Are they most concerned about cost, disability, pain, or appearance? What other concerns do they have?

Watch Your Tone

Listen to the tone of your voice. Is it high-pitched and stressed as if you are too rushed to listen? Is it loud as if you are impatient, blaming, or angry? Does your tone rise at the end of your questions or sentences? This sometimes sends a message of sarcasm or disbelief.

Even if you are explaining that you have very little time, do so in a warm tone of voice as calmly as possible.

Watch Your Body Language

Do you make eye contact or do you avoid the patient's gaze? Do you shake hands when greeting the patient or only touch them as a 'patient' not a 'person?' Do you smile or frown while speaking with them? Do you sit down or do you stand with your hand on the door handle as if they are not worth your time and you can't wait to leave?

How to Cope With Your Own Emotions

Your emotions can be a mirror of what the other person is feeling. Be curious about what you are feeling and what it can tell you about what's happening between you and your patient.

For example, when your patient is feeling anxious and desperate, you may begin to feel anxious and desperate, as well. When your patient is angry, you are likely to feel angry and want to defend yourself and/or attack the other person's position.

Of course, your emotions also reflect your own self-talk, expectations and experiences.

Many of the emotions you experience in the course of your work will be positive.

You may feel honored and grateful for the chance to be of service. You may appreciate your patients' positive emotions toward you. You may feel pride in your work.

You probably value the experience of your patients' placing their trust and confidence in you. You cherish the experience of being confident in your ability to help someone. It feels very good when you have both faith that your patient will follow your recommendations and confidence that this will lead to a successful outcome.

Think about how good it feels when you like your patient and when you enjoy what you do during your work. At times we act out of duty or in rote compliance with procedures, but most of us who enter a healthcare-related field do so because we want to help others. It is a good feeling. The more often we feel this way in our daily work, the happier and more satisfied we are.

But we are all human. We are also going to feel emotions that are more difficult, more unpleasant, and more negative.

In your training, you probably spent many hours learning about diagnosis and treatment. You learned about the physical realities of the problems your patients would have.

But were you taught that you would experience strong emotional reactions in response to your patients? Were you trained in how to respond to your emotional reactions? Few of us were.

You are human, too. You have your own emotional reactions, your own personality, genetics, biochemistry, past experiences, expectations, and knowledge or assumptions.

Emotions That Are Difficult To Handle

What are some of the most commonly experienced negative emotions?

- Hopelessness or Helplessness

- Guilt and Self-Blame

- Frustration and Anger

- Desire To Escape

Dealing with someone with a chronic illness can make you feel hopeless or helpless. You may blame yourself and feel guilty because you can't cure the problem. You may feel frustrated and angry, especially if you make unrealistic demands on yourself.

When we can't fix things, we can get angry. When other people are upset with us, we can get angry. When patients don't follow treatment recommendations, it is very easy to feel angry or frustrated.

Obviously, these feelings aren't pleasant and reinforcing. As a result, you may want to run away, emotionally or physically.

You may find yourself wanting to minimize or ignore your patients' feelings and problems—like the physician who told a patient that she should be "grateful" because the cancer treatment that caused her lymphedema "saved your life." Clearly, this response is understandable—but not helpful to the patient.

What Can You Do?

Here are some specific suggestions to help you decrease your own negative emotions.

Redefine Success

If you define success as curing lymphedema, you guarantee that you'll feel at least some of the negative emotions above—if not all! You can't "cure" lymphedema. At this time, nobody can. Your patients will not all follow your treatment recommendations. Not all of them will like or accept what you have to tell them.

So what is successful care? What can you demand and expect of yourself? What can you be proud of achieving? Consider the following:

- Stay alert for symptoms: ask, examine, and/or measure.
- Give information and/or refer to reputable sources information and/or support groups.
- Provide, or refer for, treatment to reduce symptoms and risk of complications.
- Convey respect, empathy, and concern.
- Offer hope, encouragement, and support.
- Use communications skills to better understand your patients' experience.
- Provide a listening ear and a caring heart to support patients' efforts to problem-solve.
- Help your patients move forward in the process of change, based on where they are currently in this process (see Chapter 15 for details).

Write down any additional ways in which you can succeed with your patients:

_____

_____

Don't Take It All on Your Shoulders

What do you control? What do you not control?

You control what you say and do. You control the actions you take in order to expand your knowledge, improve your expertise, and deepen your empathy and compassion. You control your responses to your thoughts and emotions. By making time to read this book you are clearly demonstrating your interest and concern.

You don't control what your patient feels. You don't control what your patient does. You don't control the choices your patient makes. You don't control the reimbursement system.

Remember, you can only be responsible for the things you directly control. You need to take full responsibility for those matters. But if you take responsibility for what's out of your control, you set yourself up for all the negative emotions discussed above.

Look Beneath the Anger

When you do feel angry, explore it. Just as you should be curious about what is behind your patient's anger, you should be curious about what is behind your own anger.

- Are you demanding the impossible?

- What thoughts and feelings are underneath, fueling the anger? Are you feeling guilty? Afraid? Hopeless? Overwhelmed?

- Are you angry because your patient requires emergency visits due to infections that could have been prevented if only they had followed your advice?

- Are you frustrated because your patients are not receiving the treatment you prescribed because Medicare or the insurance company refuses to pay? Are you spending hours on paperwork trying to reverse a "denial" by the insurance company?

See Chapter 4 for specific suggestions for dealing with anger.

Remember Your Values

Externally, there are increasing stresses on all health care professionals. Regulatory demands and documentation requirements continue to increase without increase in compensation. Demands are made to see more patients in less time and to do more with fewer resources.

You may feel stressed, harried, pressured, overworked, under appreciated, and underpaid. You may feel angry, discouraged, guilty, frustrated, or overwhelmed.

Stop for a minute right now and think about those things that may interfere with listening to your patients, with being open and responsive to them. Think about some of the negative emotions you may feel that are troublesome to you.

_____

_____

Now, stop and remember what led you to go into your profession. Think about the rewards. Think about your values. Think about what is gratifying to you and why it is worth it to take the time to improve your understanding and your communication.

_____

_____

If You Make a Mistake

Health care is not a perfect science. Treatments are not always effective or perfectly carried out. No one is omniscient, and that includes you. No one is perfect, and that includes you.

This means that, despite your best efforts, you will make mistakes. What can you do when that happens? I am not a malpractice attorney and cannot give you legal advice; however, I do sit on a quality assurance committee and have some familiarity with the research on malpractice.

In my opinion, the same factors that are tremendously important in creating a therapeutic relationship are those that can help salvage it when there has been a mistake or an unexpected treatment failure. These are:

- Caring

- Communication

- Honesty

- Listening with acceptance and respect

In the words of a respected obstetrician-gynecologist who retired after a long and successful career, *"Communicate. Communicate honestly. I never had a breath of a lawsuit – and I saw lawsuits coming out of the walls. If something went wrong, I would say, 'I'm sorry. I made a mistake. I'll do everything in my power to correct it. I understand if you're upset.' And then I'd listen."*[7]

How do you handle mistakes or failures? If you find yourself denying or hiding them, what keeps you from being honest? What keeps you from admitting mistakes to your patients, to your staff or colleagues, to yourself? Are your reasons valid? Are there better ways to handle this?

Write down the answers to these questions. Then think about what you might want to change.

_____

_____

The Next Step

Review your answers to the questions in this chapter. Think about your patients, the feelings they have, and the feelings you experience.

Identify things you want to change or improve. These are your goals. Write them in the first column of the worksheet on page 423.

Now, decide how you can use the ideas in this chapter to help you and your patients. Write specific suggestions or phrases in the second column.

Summary

I had two goals in writing this chapter. The first was to provide information that will deepen your understanding of your patients. The second was to offer suggestions that will strengthen your patient relationships and increase your effectiveness and your personal satisfaction.

You may find other portions of this book to be helpful:

- See **Sections I and II** for a more in-depth discussion of the common emotional reactions to lymphedema. For information about a specific emotional reaction, use the table of contents or index to locate relevant sections.

- I encourage you to read **Sections III, IV, and V** which cover the process of deciding to make a change, present skills that are useful in changing emotions, and discuss ways to maintain positive changes over time. You may find these skills useful both with your patients and in your personal life.

- **Chapter 22: Family and Friends** and **Chapter 25: Mental Health Professionals** may also be of interest.

I hope you find this useful, personally and professionally.

Worksheet 24-1: Actions to Improve My Effectiveness

What I Will Do or Remember to Reach My Goals											
My Goals											

Resources

About Lymphedema

Living Well With Lymphedema by Ann Ehrlich, Alma Vinjé-Harrewijn, PT, CLT and Elizabeth McMahon, PhD. Lymph Notes, 2005.

A Primer on Lymphedema by Deborah G. Kelly. Pearson Education, 2001.

Lymph Notes (www.LymphNotes.com) an online information resource and support group for persons with lymphedema, for those at risk of developing it, and for their family members and for lymphedema therapists. It also provides information about lymphedema, treatment resources, and support groups.

The National Lymphedema Network (www.lymphnet.org) is a nonprofit organization that represents lymphedema professionals and patients by providing information about lymphedema, treatment resources, and support groups.

Successful Communication

The Autonomous Patient: Ending Paternalism in Medical Care by Angela Coulter. London, England: Nuffield Trust, 2002.

"Enriching the doctor-patient relationship by inviting the patient's perspective." Delbanco TL. Ann Intern Med. 1992;116:414-418.

"The not-so-simple truth." Huff C. Hospitals & Health Networks. August 2005; 44-55.

"Assessing the effects of physician-patient interactions on the outcomes of chronic disease." Kaplan SH, Greenfield S, Ware JE. Med Care. 1989;27(suppl 3):S110-S127.

The Intelligent Patient's Guide To The Doctor-Patient Relationship: Learning How To Talk So Your Doctor Will Listen by Barbara Korsch, MD and Caroline Harding. Oxford University Press, 1997.

"Important elements of outpatient care: a comparison of patients' and physicians' opinions." Laine C, Davidoff F, Lewis CE, et al. Ann Intern Med. 1996;125:640-645.

Motivational Interviewing: Preparing People for Change, 2nd Ed by William Miller, PhD and Stephen Rollnick, PhD. Guilford Press, 2002.

Health Behavior Change: A Guide for Practitioners by Stephen Rollnick, PhD, Pip Mason, RN, and Chris Butler, MD. Churchill Livingstone, 1999.

"A 'stages of change' approach to helping patients change behavior." Zimmerman, G, Olsen, C, and Bosworth, M. American Family Physician. 2000;61:1409-1416.

Notes

1 Janice N. Cormier, MD, MPH. Private communication, August 21, 2005.

2 "Breast cancer-related lymphedema." R. M. Morrell, et al. *Mayo Clin Proc* November 2005; 80(11):1480-1484. "The reported incidence of lymphedema after standard axillary dissection can be as high as 56%... Lymphedema can be exacerbated by adjuvant radiotherapy...[T]he incidence of lymphedema has been shown to increase each year after initial breast cancer treatment." P. 1481

3 "Breast cancer-related lymphedema." R. M. Morrell, et al. *Mayo Clin Proc* November 2005; 80(11):1480-1484.

4 "Women's experiences of lymphedema." B. J. Carter. *Oncology Nursing Forum* 1997; 24(5):875-882.
Tobin MB, Lacey HF, Meyer L, Mortimer PS: The psychological morbidity of breast cancer-related arm swelling. Psychological morbidity of lymphoedema. Cancer 72(11): 3248-3252, 1993.
"Single center experiences in chronic lymphedema: What we learned through clinical analysis." E. Kim and B. Lee. National Lymphedema Network newsletter, *Lymph Link* Oct-Dec 2004 issue; 16(4):4.
Velanovich V, Szymanski W: Quality of life of breast cancer patients with lymphedema. Am J Surg 177(3): 184-187, 1999.
Kornblith AB, Ligibel J: Psychosocial and sexual functioning of survivors of breast cancer. Semin Oncol 30(6): 799-813, 2003.
"Women's experiences of lymphedema" by B. J. Carter. *Oncology Nursing Forum* 1997; 24(5):875-882.
"Quality of life and a symptom cluster associated with breast cancer

treatment-related lymphedema" by S. H. Ridner. *Supportive Care in Cancer*, 2005 Nov; 13(11:904-911. Epub2005 Apr 6.

5   "Lymphedema and Quality of Life in Survivors of Early-Stage Breast Cancer" by S Beaulac, L McNair, T Scott, W LaMorte, and M Kava- nah. Arch Surg, 2002, 137: 1253-1257.
    "Psychosocial benefits of Postmastectomy lymphedema therapy" by B. R. Mirolo, et al. Cancer Nursing, 1995; 18(3):197-205.

6   "Assessing the effects of physician-patient interactions on the out- comes of chronic disease." Kaplan SH, Greenfield S, Ware JE. *Med Care*. 1989;27(suppl 3):S110-S127.

7   Edmund B. McMahon, MD. Private communication, June 23, 2005.

For Mental Health Professionals

This chapter is for mental health professionals who are treating people with lymphedema. It covers:

- Information about lymphedema and its impact on patients
- Therapeutic issues likely to arise in psychotherapy with lymphedema patients
- Sources of more information

This information may also be helpful for treating people with other chronic medical conditions.

What Is Lymphedema?

Lymphedema is a swelling (or edema) in tissues that results from an imbalance between the rate of lymphatic fluid creation and the body's ability to move this fluid out of the body tissues, transport it to the lymph nodes to be cleaned, and return it to the blood circulatory system. See Appendix A and the references for more information.

The two most common forms of lymphedema in the United States are primary and secondary. Primary lymphedema is hereditary and frequently develops during adolescence, although it can appear at any age.

Secondary lymphedema results from an injury, medical treatment, or other medical conditions. The most common causes of secondary lymphedema are diagnostic or treatment procedures for cancer: biopsy, lymph node removal, radiation, etc. Secondary lymphedema affects an estimated 20-40% of cancer survivors. Lymphedema can also be caused by chronic venous insufficiency, lipedema, obesity, or paralysis.

Lymphedema can worsen other medical problems. For example, either primary or secondary lymphedema can cause or exacerbate problems with muscles and joints.

Lymphedema is a chronic condition. It may be controlled by a combination of treatment and self-care, but currently there is no cure. If it is not well controlled, it is a progressive and degenerative condition.

What Does It Mean To Have Lymphedema?

Lymphedema affects a person's life in many ways. People with lymphedema face many physical, emotional, social, and financial challenges.

Lymphedema Can Be a Lonely, Isolating Condition

Most people have never heard of lymphedema. They have no understanding of the lymphatic system and don't understand the serious, demanding nature of the condition. This makes it hard to discuss lymphedema with others and to find sympathy, support, treatment, and practical advice.

People with lymphedema are less likely to socialize due to a variety of factors including self-consciousness related to the deformity caused by the swelling, physical discomfort, and decreased mobility due to the physical effects of the lymphedema.

Lymphedema Is a Serious Condition

Tissues affected by lymphedema are constantly at risk for infections. Any break in the skin can result in rapidly spreading cellulitis that can be life threatening. Treatment for these infections may require hospitalization and IV antibiotics.

Lymphedema can be disabling, especially in combination with other medical conditions like obesity, orthopedic, or circulatory problems. Poorly controlled lymphedema will permanently damage the tissues and skin as the swelling increases to the point that the skin hangs in folds.

Lymphedema Is a Chronic Condition

Lymphedema must be actively treated and managed for the rest of the patient's life. It can never be forgotten. It can never be ignored. Lymphedema interferes with simple pleasures and activities that most of us take for granted.

Because of the danger of infection, the patient must always be alert for anything that may break or puncture the skin. People get tired of the daily self-management regimen which can feel like "*an ongoing battle.*"

Lymphedema Affects Relationships

Lymphedema can place significant stress on the relationship. In response to the stress of chronic illness, relationships change. They may either become weaker or stronger; they do not stay the same.

Lymphedema Is a Progressive Condition

Left untreated, lymphedema is a progressive condition where the skin of the affected area deteriorates and hardens (becomes fibrotic or develops fibrosis). Effective treatment and self-management will slow or halt this progression.

Lymphedema is more effectively controlled in the early stages. Once fibrosis develops, it makes treatment more difficult and severe, life-threatening infections occur more frequently.

As time passes, it can be easy for the person with lymphedema to become discouraged and to give up on the daily self-management. However, not doing daily self-care causes the condition to worsen and then more intensive treatment may be needed.

Lymphedema Care is Expensive

Lymphedema care involves a combination of periodic professional treatment and daily self-management. Frequently it is up to the patient to locate and arrange lymphedema treatment. The frequency of professional treatment varies with the patient's condition and ability to afford treatment.

There is a shortage of qualified lymphedema therapists, making it hard to find treatment. Some facilities hire therapists who have not met the national training standards. Treatment by a poorly trained therapist may not be effective and can waste precious visits paid for by insurance.

Self-management for effective lymphedema care involves self-massage, specialized exercises, compression garments or bandages, and skin care. In some cases, two or more hours each day may need to be devoted to lymphedema self-management. Compression garments are expensive and must be replaced periodically. Some bandaging supplies are only used once; others are reusable but must be replaced frequently.

Most healthcare reimbursement programs do not cover the full cost of lymphedema care. Many do not cover the cost of compression garments or bandages, which can be quite expensive. Some limit the number of treatments allowed per year.

As a result, money needs to be spent on lymphedema treatment that would otherwise be available for other uses. Meanwhile, the person may be earning less money or unable to work because of lymphedema-related disability.

Lymphedema patients spend time and energy fighting for reimbursement. Having a chronic condition, such as lymphedema, makes it more difficult to obtain or change health insurance coverage.

Lymphedema Can Be Disfiguring

The fluid build-up can cause limbs to be swollen, heavy, and uncomfortable. Clothes may no longer fit. If one leg is affected it may be necessary to buy two different sizes of shoes to accommodate the difference.

A limb can easily swell to more than twice its normal size and this swelling can be visible to others. Severe swelling, particularly of the leg, can make the tissues hang in folds. Severe swelling of the hand can interfere with activities requiring finger motions such as writing, typing, eating, or food preparation.

Special compression garments should be worn at all times. Usually a knit compression garment is worn during the day while active. Bandages or a specialized compression garment is worn at other times. These requirements make wearing standard clothing difficult or impossible.

People with secondary lymphedema may have additional appearance issues related to the cause of their lymphedema. For example, if they have lymphedema as a result of a mastectomy, accidental burns, or severe scarring.

Lymphedema Can Be Painful

The lymph in the swollen tissues can press against nerves causing pain, tingling, and/or burning sensations. The weight of the swelling and the effect of the excess lymphatic fluid on joints can cause or exacerbate orthopedic problems resulting in pain.

Lymphedema Can Be a Reminder of Its Cause

Having to deal with secondary lymphedema every day makes it harder for the person to go on with life and put the past medical trauma behind them. Some breast cancer survivors with lymphedema say that the lymphedema is harder for them to deal with than the breast cancer.

Lymphedema Patients Can Feel Angry, Betrayed, or Abandoned

Lingering anger at the medical profession is a common problem for people with secondary lymphedema caused by medical treatment. Patients often feel alone and abandoned.

Many report that they were never told of the possible risk of lymphedema before agreeing to the medical procedure that caused it. Others report that they were informed of the possibility, but were not advised on ways to avoid developing it.

Support networks may be mobilized during the acute, dramatic crisis of cancer. After the triumph of surviving cancer has been achieved and celebrated, the level of support may drop drastically. Cancer survivors may then be left to cope alone with a condition requiring lifelong daily care. Cancer is discussed in the media. Lymphedema rarely is. Patients can feel bereft, isolated, and even ashamed.

Once someone develops lymphedema, it may take some time and several doctors before the condition is diagnosed. Primary lymphedema, in particular, may be present for years before being accurately diagnosed.

Many people also report that after they are diagnosed with lymphedema, their healthcare professionals had little help to offer them. Lymphedema treatment may be hard to find and/or located a considerable distance away.

Lymphedema Affects Quality of Life

Studies of women after breast cancer treatment have compared those who developed lymphedema with those who did not. A consistent finding from this body of literature is that those with lymphedema have more emotional distress.

Not surprisingly, these women report a lower quality of life (QOL) than those without lymphedema. Quality of life scores may drop to their lowest level immediately after diagnosis and during initial, intensive lymphedema treatment. Scores may then rebound or even surpass pretreatment levels after completing intensive lymphedema treatment.[1] Among lymphedema sufferers, women who consistently followed their self-care plan were more likely to report improved QOL scores.[2]

However, in general, quality of life levels in breast cancer survivors with lymphedema are below the levels of those survivors without lymphedema.[3] In other words, this condition continues to carry a psychological burden.[4]

Issues Relevant To Psychotherapy

Sections I and II of this book discuss the emotional challenges that commonly accompany lymphedema. Reading these will give you both a better understanding of what lymphedema entails and a deeper empathy for your clients.

A person may be seeking psychotherapy specifically to focus on one or more of the emotional challenges covered earlier in this book or they may be seeking counseling for another issue entirely.

In either case, you may want to be alert for certain issues discussed below:

- Co-occurring psychological conditions
- Medical issues
- Treatment approaches
- Therapist issues.

Possible Co-Occurring Psychological Conditions

Be alert to a possible depressive disorder. This is important for two reasons. First, depression can interfere with emotional and physical self-care. Second, very effective psychotherapeutic and psychopharmacologic treatments for depression exist.

Studies of people post-cancer-treatment and of people with chronic illnesses find that a significant percentage of them show and/or report symptoms of depression. The incidence of depression may be higher in people coping with lymphedema, especially if they experience pain.

Depression is a comorbid disabling syndrome that affects approximately 15% to 25% of cancer patients and is believed to affect men and women with cancer equally.[5] The Lance Armstrong Foundation polled 1,020 cancer survivors, 70% of respondents said they had to deal with depression as a result of their cancer, within this group 88% said they had some level of difficulty dealing with the issue yet 78% *did not* seek out the services of a counselor, social worker, psychologist or psychiatrist.[6]

Be alert to the possible presence of one or more anxiety disorders or related disorders:

- Depression makes anxiety more likely. The reverse is also true: anxiety makes depression more likely.

- Visible physical conditions make body image problems and social anxiety more likely.

- Factors such as stress, trauma, serious illness, and uncertainty about the future all make anxiety and anxiety disorders more likely.

- The person who has one anxiety problem is likely to have, or to develop, other anxiety problems in addition.

Be alert to the possibility of relationship issues. Lymphedema can stress marital and family relationships.[7] However, relationships can also be strengthened.[8] However, a certain number of relationships are weakened and may end.[9]

In patients with primary lymphedema, an inherited condition, issues of anger toward parents and/or guilt or responsibility toward children may need to be addressed. If a couple wishes to conceive children together and one partner has primary lymphedema, a referral for genetic counseling may be appropriate.

Relevant Medical Issues

Be alert to the effects of past illnesses.

- Was secondary lymphedema caused by cancer-related diagnostic or treatment procedures? Lymphedema is a common consequence of the surgical treatment of cancer, especially breast, gynecologic, genitourinary cancers, melanoma, and sarcoma.[10]

- Was lymphedema caused by a traumatic accident or injury?

- What other sequelae of these events are present?

- What is the medical prognosis?

- How might these factors be affecting the person physically and emotionally?

Be aware of possible psychological effects of any medications.

Be alert to the possible presence and effects of other chronic illnesses, such as diabetes or venous insufficiency. Encourage good medical care and control of these conditions.

Be alert to the possible presence and effects of other medical/psychological problems, such as obesity and/or eating disorders. Encourage a healthy lifestyle.

Develop at least some understanding of lymphedema and its treatment.

- Be familiar with common lymphedema self-management recommendations. See **Living Well With Lymphedema** for details.

- Ask about the specific recommendations your patient has received.

- Encourage and support full implementation of an effective self-management program.

- Explore factors that interfere with effective care of the lymphedema.

Issues Relevant To Treatment Approaches

In many ways, each treatment is unique because the people involved are unique. Each psychotherapist is an individual with differences in personality, style, training, experience, knowledge, expertise, and resources for expert supervision and further training. Every person seeking psychotherapy is an individual with differences in personality, history, living situation, knowledge, skills, and resources for therapy.

The suggestions given throughout this book draw from various sources including (in alphabetical order) behavioral psychotherapies, client-centered psychotherapy, cognitive psychotherapies, dialectical behavior therapy, existential psychotherapy, Gestalt psychotherapy, and psychodynamic psychotherapies, among others.

In making treatment recommendations, I have sometimes had a choice between treatments with research support and treatments with no (or less) research support. In these instances, I have tried to select or emphasize treatments that appear to have the strongest empirical evidence for their effectiveness.

Throughout the book, I have given coping tips, presented self-help skills, and included resources for more information about relevant topics. These have been drawn, in part, from my best understanding of the current research literature and, in part, from clinical experience.

Therapist Issues

Working with lymphedema patients might also raise issues for you as a therapist. Spend some time exploring possible countertransference or reactions that might interfere with your treatment of people with lymphedema. Ask yourself:

- Do I become uneasy when faced with visible physical differences?

- Am I frightened or depressed when I consider the prospect of having a lifelong, chronic condition?

- Do I feel helpless or uncomfortable with patients who have a medical condition that cannot be cured?

- Are there issues from my past or in my present that might interfere with working with these problems?

- What problems could occur if I treat someone with lymphedema?

- What worst outcomes could I imagine? How could I prevent them?

Write down your answers and any other thoughts that occur to you as you read.

_____

_____

What exactly will you do to change your unhelpful thoughts and emotional responses? While working on changing, how will you monitor your thoughts and ensure that they do not interfere with helping your client? What would be the earliest warning signs of problems? What will you do?

_____

_____

With whom can you discuss these issues without breaching patient-therapist confidentiality?

_____

Stay within the limits of your training, your licensure, and your expertise. Actively seek out consultation, supervision, and/or additional training as needed.

Chapter 25: For Health Care Professionals also has information that is relevant to creating and sustaining a positive therapeutic relationship.

Summary

Providing psychotherapy to someone who has lymphedema can be deeply satisfying. You can be witness to, and partner in, the development of life-changing skills.

Overcoming the emotional challenges of a chronic condition will result in increased happiness and self-confidence. It also results in a deepened appreciation of the positives in one's life and one's self.

Grappling with issues such as self-worth in the face of adversity can increase wisdom, maturity, understanding, and compassion. Dealing with others' reactions can develop courage, social skills, and self-confidence. Learning and practicing the skills that allow one to care for one's self, emotionally and physically, can be enormously freeing.

As a psychotherapist, it is an honor to help someone achieve these changes. I hope you, and those you help, find the information in this book useful.

You may find Chapter 24: **For Healthcare Professionals** and Chapter 22: **For Family and Friends** to be helpful as well.

Resources

The books listed below are written for the psychotherapist. This is not a comprehensive listing of all treatments manuals or treatment approaches to these problems. My emphasis is on books that present treatment approaches that have research evidence of effectiveness.

At the end of most chapters in this book, you will find self-help books and client treatment manuals listed in the **Resources** section.

Reviews of Empirically-Supported Treatments

These two volumes comprehensively review the psychosocial and pharma-cological treatments for which there is documented effectiveness. Together they cover treatments for agoraphobia, body dysmorphic disorder, eating disorders, hypochondriasis, generalized anxiety, obesity, obsessive-compul-sive disorder, panic, phobias, post-traumatic stress, social anxiety, somatiza-tion, and substance abuse.

Clinical Handbook of Psychological Disorders, Third Edition: A Step-by-Step Treatment Manual edited by David Barlow, PhD Guilford Press, 2001.

A Guide To Treatments That Work, Second Edition edited by Peter Nathan, PhD and Jack Gorman, MD. Oxford University Press, 2002.

Research Findings

The best way to stay current with the research is by reading the peer-reviewed psychology and psychiatry journals. An additional resource is the American Psychological Association's "web-based compendium of psychological research" that presents research findings, based on well-designed studies, with immediate practical value and application. See www.psychologymatters.org.

Anger Management

Anger Management: The Complete Treatment Guidebook for Practitioners by Howard Kassinove, PhD and Raymond Tafrate, PhD. Impact Publishers, 2002.

Anxiety Disorders

Anxiety Disorders and Phobias: A Cognitive Perspective by Aaron Beck, MD, Gary Emery, PhD, and Ruth Greenberg, PhD. Basic Books Reprint Edition, 1990.

Treatment Plans and Interventions for Depression and Anxiety Disorders by Robert Leahy, PhD and Stephen Holland, PsyD. Guilford Press, 2000.

The Anxiety Disorders Association of America (www.adaa.org) is a nonprofit organization providing information about the diagnosis and treatment of anxiety disorders.

Body Dysmorphic Disorder and/or Body Image Problems

The Broken Mirror: Understanding and Treating Body Dysmorphic Disorder by Katharine Phillips, MD. Oxford University Press, 1998.

Body Image: A Handbook of Theory, Research, and Clinical Practice edited by Thomas Cash, PhD and Thomas Pruzinsky, PhD. Guilford Press, 2004.

Depression

Cognitive Therapy of Depression by Aaron Beck, MD, A. John Rush, MD, Brian Shaw, PhD, and Gary Emery, PhD. Guilford Press, 1979.

Treatment Plans and Interventions for Depression and Anxiety Disorders by Robert Leahy, PhD and Stephen Holland, PsyD. Guilford Press, 2000.

Eating Disorders and/or Obesity

Eating Disorders and Obesity, Second Edition: A Comprehensive Handbook edited by Christopher Fairburn and Kelly Brownell. Guilford Press, 2002.

Overcoming Eating Disorders: A Cognitive-Behavioral Treatment for Bulimia Nervosa and Binge-Eating, Therapist Guide by W. Stewart Agras and Robin Apple. Academic Press, 1999.

Cognitive-Behavioral Treatment of Obesity: A Clinician's Guide by Zafra Cooper, PhD, Christopher Fairburn, MD, and Deborah Hawker, PhD Guilford Press, 2004.

Generalized Anxiety Disorder

Mastery of Your Anxiety and Worry, Therapist Guide by Richard Zinbarg, PhD, Michelle Craske, PhD, and David Barlow, PhD Oxford University Press, 1992.

Generalized Anxiety Disorder: Advances in Research and Practice edited by Richard Heimberg, PhD, Cynthia Turk, PhD, and Douglas Mennin, PhD Guilford Press, 2004.

Hypochondriasis

Health Anxiety: Research and Clinical Perspectives on Hypochondriasis and Related Conditions edited by Gordon Asmundson, Steven Taylor, and Brian Cox. John Wiley, 2001.

Marital Therapy

Acceptance And Change in Couple Therapy: A Therapist's Guide to Transforming Relationships by Neil Jacobson, PhD and Andrew Christensen, PhD W. W. Norton, 1998.

Clinical Handbook of Marital Therapy, Third Edition edited by Alan Gurman, PhD and Neil Jacobson, PhD Guilford Press, 2002.

Cognitive Behavioral Marital Therapy by Donald Baucom, PhD and Norman Epstein, PhD Brunner/Mazel, 1990.

Motivational Interviewing

Health Behavior Change: A Guide for Practitioners by Stephen Rollnick, PhD, Pip Mason, RN, and Chris Butler, MD. Churchill Livingstone, 1999.

Motivational Interviewing: Preparing People for Change, 2nd Edition by William Miller, PhD and Stephen Rollnick, PhD. Guilford Press, 2002.

Obsessive-Compulsive Disorder

Cognitive-Behavioral Therapy for OCD by David Clark, PhD Guilford Press, 2004.

Pain and Chronic Pain

Cognitive Therapy for Chronic Pain: A Step-By-Step Guide by Beverly Thorn, PhD Guilford Press, 2004.

Pain Management Psychotherapy: A Practical Guide by Bruce Eimer, PhD and Arthur Freeman, EdD. John Wiley and Sons, 1998.

Panic Disorder With or Without Agoraphobia

Mastery of Your Anxiety and Panic, MAP-3, Therapist Guide by Michelle Craske, PhD, Martin Antony, PhD, and David Barlow, PhD Oxford University Press, 2000.

Post-Traumatic Stress Disorder

Overcoming Post-Traumatic Stress Disorder—Therapist Protocol: A Cognitive-Behavioral Exposure-Based Protocol for the Treatment of PTSD and Other Anxiety Disorders by Larry Smyth, PhD 2002.

Specific Phobias

Mastery of Your Specific Phobia, Therapist Guide by Martin Antony, PhD, Michelle Craske, PhD, and David Barlow, PhD Oxford University Press, 1995.

Substance Abuse

Cognitive Therapy of Substance Abuse by Aaron Beck, MD, Fred Wright, EdD, Cory Newman, PhD, and Bruce Liese, PhD. Guilford Press, 1993.

Seeking Safety: A Treatment Manual for PTSD and Substance Abuse by Lisa Najavits. Guilford Press, 2001.

Notes

1   "Psychosocial benefits of Postmastectomy lymphedema therapy" by B. R. Mirolo, et al. *Cancer Nursing*, 1995; 18(3):197-205.

2   "Lymphedema and Quality of Life in Survivors of Early-Stage Breast Cancer" by S Beaulac, L McNair, T Scott, W LaMorte, and M Kavanah. Arch Surg, 2002, 137: 1253-1257.

3   Sheila Ridner, PhD, RN. Private communication, August 13, 2005. "Quality of life and a symptom cluster associated with breast cancer treatment-related lymphedema" by S. H. Ridner. *Supportive Care in Cancer*, 2005 Nov; 13(11:904-911. Epub2005 Apr 6.

4   "Women's experiences of lymphedema." B. J. Carter. *Oncology Nursing Forum* 1997; 24(5):875-882.
Tobin MB, Lacey HF, Meyer L, Mortimer PS: The psychological morbidity of breast cancer-related arm swelling. Psychological morbidity of lymphoedema. Cancer 72(11): 3248-3252, 1993.
"Single center experiences in chronic lymphedema: What we learned through clinical analysis." E. Kim and B. Lee. National Lymphedema Network newsletter, *Lymph Link* Oct-Dec 2004 issue; 16(4):4.
Velanovich V, Szymanski W: Quality of life of breast cancer patients with lymphedema. Am J Surg 177(3): 184-187, 1999.
Kornblith AB, Ligibel J: Psychosocial and sexual functioning of survivors of breast cancer. Semin Oncol 30(6): 799-813, 2003.
"Women's experiences of lymphedema" by B. J. Carter. *Oncology Nursing Forum* 1997; 24(5):875-882.

5   Data from www.cancer.gov/cancertopics/pdq/supportivecare/depression/healthprofessional accessed on July 18, 2005.

6   LIVESTRONG Poll Fact Sheet by the Lance Armstrong Foundation, November 30, 2004.

7   "Psychiatric consultation for women undergoing rehabilitation for upper-extremity lymphedema following breast cancer treatment" by S. Passik, M. Newman, M. Brennan, and J. Holland. *Journal of Pain and Symptom Management* 1993; 8(4):226-233.
"Lymphedema: Strategies for management" by S. R. Cohen, D. K. Payne, and R. S. Tunkel. *Cancer*, Supplement August 15, 2001; 92(4):980-987.

8   Kornblith AB, Ligibel J: Psychosocial and sexual functioning of survivors of breast cancer. Semin Oncol 30(6): 799-813, 2003.

9   "Psychopathology and Marital Satisfaction: The Importance of Evaluating Both Partners," Mark A. Whisman, et al. Journal of Consulting and Clinical Psychology, Vol. 72, No. 5.

10 Janice N. Cormier, MD, MPH. Private communication, August 21, 2005.

About Lymphedema

This appendix explains lymphedema, its causes, complications, and treatment very briefly. For more detail, see the resources under Resources.

What is Lymphedema?

Lymphedema (or lymphoedema) is swelling (edema) that results from an imbalance between the rate at which lymphatic fluid is created and the body's ability to move this fluid out of the tissues. Excess lymphatic fluid, or lymph, accumulates in the skin and around the underlying structures. Swelling due to lymphedema is not discolored like the swelling caused by bruising or bleeding. Trapped lymphatic fluid is rich in protein which increases the risk of infection.

Primary lymphedema is an inherited condition that can appear at any age and in either sex. Primary lymphedema is more common in females than males and most commonly appears during adolescence affecting the feet and legs.

Secondary or acquired lymphedema accounts for more than 90% of the lymphedema cases in the US.[1] This condition caused by damage to the lymphatic system or interference with its action as explained below.

What is Lymph?

Lymph, or lymphatic fluid, is a colorless fluid found in all body tissues. Lymph acts as a garbage collector and removes debris including dead blood cells, pathogens, toxins, cancer cells, and protein molecules, as part of the lymphatic system.

Blood is made up of blood plasma that carries red blood cells, white blood cells, and platelets in suspension. Plasma flows out of the capillaries and becomes tissue fluid, carrying oxygen, nutrients, and hormones into the cells. Tissue fluid flows out of the cells again carrying waste.

Most of the tissue fluid flows back into the circulatory system and becomes plasma again. About one tenth of the tissue fluid carries waste proteins that are too large to reenter the cardiovascular system. This fluid is known as lymph and is normally removed by the lymphatic system.

What is the Lymphatic System?

The lymphatic system is part of the immune system that keeps us healthy by destroying cancer cells and pathogens. The lymphatic system:

- Removes waste and excess fluid from tissues and returns proteins and fluid to the cardiovascular system.

- Circulates *lymphocytes*, white blood cells that make antibodies and help destroy invading organisms.

- Absorbs fats and fat-soluble vitamins in the digestive system.

The lymphatic system has several parts:

- **Lymphatic capillaries** are tiny tubes where lymph enters the lymphatic system. About 70% of the lymphatic capillaries are located in or just under the skin, the other 30% are found around internal organs.

- **Pre-collectors, collectors, trunks, and ducts** are the progressively larger vessels of the lymphatic system that collect lymph, process it through the lymph nodes, and return the processed lymph to the cardiovascular system.

- **Lymph nodes** are bean shaped nodules connect to the lymphatic trunks where lymph is filtered and processed by lymphocytes. Lymph nodes may become enlarged while fighting an infection; what many people call 'swollen glands' are enlarged lymph nodes in the neck.

How Does the Lymphatic System Work?

Lymph from the tissues flows into the lymphatic capillaries. These capillaries flow into progressively larger pre-collectors and collectors that flow into lymph nodes. The lymph nodes clean the lymph. The lymphatic trunks carry the output of the lymph nodes to the lymphatic ducts which return the fluid to the cardiovascular system.

Lymph nodes are located throughout the body. The larger nodes are located in clusters: cervical nodes along either side of the neck, axillary nodes in each armpit, and inguinal nodes in the groin.

Lymph from the body flows upwards and reenters the cardiovascular system at the base of the neck, in an area known as the terminus. The upper right quarter of the body drains on the right side and the other three quarters of the body, including both legs, drains on the left side.

The heart acts as a pump for the cardiovascular system. The lymphatic system does not have a central pump and instead relies on the pumping action of the large muscles and joints together with contractions of the smooth muscles that make up the walls of lymphatic trunks.

What Causes Lymphedema?

There are many conditions that can cause lymphedema and one person may have a combination of these conditions. Each of these causes interferes with the flow of lymph in some way, either by damaging the lymphatic system or disabling the pumping mechanisms that make it work.

Primary lymphedema is an inherited condition linked to abnormal development of the lymphatic vessels. This may include the congenital absence of lymphatic vessels or lymphatic vessels that are fewer in number and smaller than usual.

Secondary lymphedema results from some form of interference with the normal functioning of the lymphatic system such as:

- Skin damage, which destroys many small lymphatic vessels, or large areas of scar tissue where lymphatic vessels are slow to re-grow. This damage may result from physical trauma, burns, radiation, surgery, etc.

- Lymph node or lymphatic vessel damage, removal, or blockage due to an accident, medical procedure, or infection. The diagnosis and treatment of some cancers includes lymph node removal (section), or lymph node biopsy, a procedure in which parts of one or more lymph nodes are removed.

- Fat accumulation under the skin due to obesity or lipedema. Lymphatic vessels in the skin drain through the layer of fat under the skin. As this fat layer becomes thicker and denser, it blocks the flow of lymph and decreases the lymph pumping effect of muscle movements.

- Inactivity, muscle damage, or paralysis decreases or eliminates the pumping action of the large muscles and joints that normally stimulates the drainage of lymph.

- Circulatory problems such as chronic venous insufficiency (CVI) and other conditions that cause inflammation may cause or contribute to lymphedema by overloading the lymphatic system with excess fluid. Over time, tissue changes due to the combination of conditions damage the lymphatic capillaries.

- Filariasis is caused by parasitic worms (filariae) that block the lymphatic vessels. Filariasis is a tropical disease spread by mosquitoes.

Anyone with one or more of these conditions is at risk for developing lymphedema.

Many cases of secondary lymphedema result from cancer treatment. Lymphedema is a common consequence of the surgical treatment of cancer, especially:

- Upper extremity lymphedema resulting from removing the lymph nodes in the armpits (axillary node dissection) as part of the treatment for breast cancer (mastectomy) or melanoma.

- Lower extremity lymphedema resulting from removing pelvic lymph nodes as part of the treatment for melanoma, sarcomas, gynecological, prostate, penile, and bladder cancers.

How Common is Lymphedema?

The World Health Organization estimates that 170 million people have secondary lymphedema. This includes 120 million cases of lymphatic filariasis, implying about 50 million people with secondary lymphedema from other causes. Lymphedema affects about 3 to 5 million people in the US including about 20-40% of cancer survivors.

What Are Complications of Lymphedema?

Complications of lymphedema can include:

*   Infections of the tissues and the stagnant lymphatic fluid including cellulitis or erysipelas. These infections can be fast spreading and life threatening; repeated bouts may lead to chronic infections.

*   Orthopedic problems with muscles and joints caused by the excess weight and the effect of the lymphatic fluid on the joints. These problems are potentially disabling.

*   Tissue and skin changes including hardening and thickening of the skin and the flow of lymph through the skin. Untreated lymphedema can lead to lymphangiosarcoma, a rare but deadly form of cancer.

How is Lymphedema Treated?

Lymphedema treatment involves a combination of professional therapy and self-management or home care. *Complete Decongestive Therapy (CDT)* is the most widely accepted therapy and includes:

*   **Manual lymph drainage** (MLD) is a specialized form of massage that gently stimulates the flow of lymph and reduces swelling.

*   **Compression techniques** to prevent additional swelling including bandaging and specialized compression garments.

*   **Exercise** to stimulate the flow of lymph through the motion of muscles and joints.

*   **Skin Care** to minimize skin deterioration that cause breaks in the skin and increase the risk of infection.

These treatments are provided by a qualified lymphedema therapist who also teaches the patient a self-management regime to be carried out at home on a daily basis. Self-management procedures include self-massage, compression with specialized garments or bandages, specialized exercises, skin care procedures, and precautionary measures.

Why is Treatment Important?

Treatment is essential to minimize the swelling, minimize the likelihood of other complications, and slow the progression of skin and tissue deterioration. Although some tissue changes can be reversed through treatment, it is much safer to start treatment early and avoid tissue changes.

Resources

Living Well With Lymphedema by Ann Ehrlich, Alma Vinjé-Harrewijn, PT, CLT and Elizabeth McMahon, PhD. Lymph Notes, 2005.

A Primer on Lymphedema by Deborah G. Kelly. Pearson Education, 2001.

Notes

1   Janice N. Cormier, MD, **Secondary Lymphedema**, presentation at the 1st International NLN Patient Summit August 18-20, 2005

Index

About the Author

Elizabeth McMahon, PhD is a clinical psychologist with more than 25 years of experience helping patients, many of whom have chronic medical conditions. She became interested in lymphedema while looking for resources for a family member.

Dr. McMahon received her BA in Psychology from Earlham College and her PhD in Clinical Psychology from Case Western Reserve University. She works in the outpatient psychiatry department of Kaiser Permanente in California where she provides individual and group therapy, supervises psychology residents, helps develop best practice guidelines, and serves on the clinical review and quality assurance committees. She is a coauthor of **Living Well With Lymphedema** (Lymph Notes, 2005).

Printed in the United States
42768LVS00004B/49-51